MAKE IT SAFE!

A FAMILY CAREGIVER'S HOME SAFETY ASSESSMENT GUIDE FOR SUPPORTING ELDERS@HOME

Companion Workbook

RAE A. STONEHOUSE

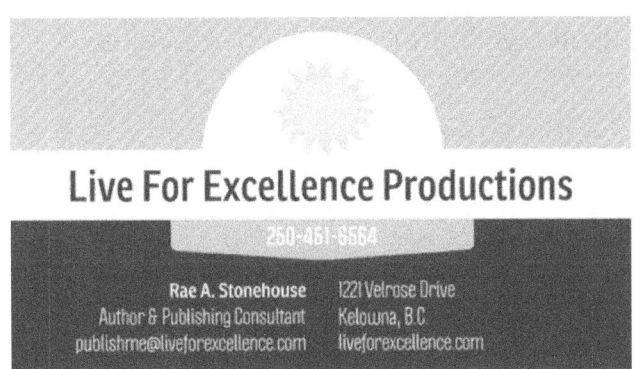

Copyright © 2020 by Rae A. Stonehouse

All rights reserved.

No part of this book may be reproduced in any form or by any electronic or mechanical means, including information storage and retrieval systems, without written permission from the author, except for the use of brief quotations in a book review.

Disclaimer: The publisher and the author are providing this book and its contents on "as is" basis and make no representations or warranties of any kind with respect to this book or its contents. The publisher and the author disclaim all such representations and warranties, including but not limited to warranties of healthcare for a particular purpose. In addition, the publisher and author assume no responsibility for errors, inaccuracies, omissions, or any other inconsistencies herein

Do your own research: The content of this book is intended to be used and must be used for informational purposes only. It is very important to do your own assessments before investing in renovations or purchasing safety equipment based on your own personal circumstances. You should independently research and verify any information provided in this book and wish to act upon.
This publication is meant as a source of valuable information for the reader, however it is not meant as a substitute for direct expert assistance. If such level of assistance is required, the services of a competent professional should be sought. The publisher and the author make no guarantees concerning the level of success you may experience by following the advice and strategies contained in this book and you accept the results will differ with each individual.

Print- ISBN: 978-1-7771565-5-8

Live for Excellence Productions
1221 Velrose Drive
Kelowna, B.C., Canada
V1X 6R7
https://liveforexcellence.com

This page has been intentionally left blank.

Contents

Introduction 13

Chapter One: Home Safety Overview 15

Introducing the 3 As of Personal safety... Awareness, Assessment and Action. 15

Chapter Two: Home Safety - Indoors General 19

    Safety Assessment Question: Is house clean & tidy? 20

    Safety Assessment Question: Is the home safe for a professional caregiver to visit the home? 20

    Safety Assessment Question: Are emergency numbers posted? 21

    Safety Assessment Question: Is there a designated danger zone in the home to store hazardous chemicals or products? 21

    Safety Assessment Question: Is there good lighting in stairways & hallways? 22

    Safety Assessment Question: Does every room have proper lighting, including walk-in closets? 22

    Safety Assessment Question: Are light switches installed at the top and bottom of staircases? 23

    Safety Assessment Question: Are bookshelves anchored to walls to prevent toppling over? ... 23

    Safety Assessment Questions: Is a smoke and carbon monoxide detector present? 23

    Safety Assessment Question: Are there any wheeled swivel chairs in the home? 24

    Safety Assessment Question: Do bedrooms or bathrooms have locks that can be released should an elder lock themselves in? 24

    Safety Assessment Question: Are doorways and halls wide enough for an elder to navigate with a wheelchair or walker? 25

    Safety Assessment Question: Are cordless phones within easy reach of the elder? 25

    Safety Assessment Questions: Is the furniture stable? 25

    Safety Assessment Question: Are furniture cushion levels at the right level to allow the elder to easily sit down? 26

    Safety Assessment Question: Are electrical cords or cables exposed in a way that could be a trip hazard? 26

    Safety Assessment Question: Are there any barriers to creating a safe home? 26

    Safety Assessment Question: Are bed rails required for the elder sleeping safety? 27

    Safety Assessment Question: Is the elder's bed at a level that allows them to place their feet on the floor when attempting to stand up from the bed? 27

    Safety Assessment Question: Is the elder's clothing safe? 27

Safety Assessment Question: Does the home have an adequate heating system or does the elder use the stove or oven to provide heat? 28

Safety Assessment Question: Have you developed an escape route in case of fire and a fire safety plan? 28

Safety Assessment Question: If the elder uses a space heater, is it placed well away from flammable substances and materials? 28

Safety Assessment Question: Is there any evidence of leaks in the home as evidenced by water stains on a ceiling or an interior wall? 29

Safety Assessment Question: Do you have a first aid kit and know where it is? 29

Miscellaneous Safety Measures: 29

Safety Devices: 31

Safety Suggestions 33

Chapter Three: Assessing Fall Hazards 35

Safety Assessment Question: Do the steps of the stairs have a non-skid surface? 35

Safety Assessment Question: Are there solid handrails on both sides of the stairway? 35

Safety Assessment Question: Are pets underfoot? 35

Safety Assessment Question: Are household pathways clear? 36

Safety Assessment Question: Does the elder wear anti-slip footwear within the house? 36

Safety Assessment Question: Are there grade changes at entrances or between flooring changes? 37

Safety Assessment Question: Do door sills present a potential tripping hazard? 37

Safety Assessment Question: Is there any clutter on the stairs? 37

Safety Assessment Question: Is the elder able to climb and descend stairs easily or with difficulty? 38

Safety Assessment Question: Are there any small furniture items that could be a trip hazard? 38

Safety Assessment Question: Are the home's high-traffic areas clear of obstacles? 38

Safety Assessment Question: If you use floor wax, do you use the non-skid kind? 39

Chapter Four: Home Safety - Hallways & Stairwells 41

Safety Assessment Question: Are household pathways clear? 41

Safety Assessment Question: Do the steps of your stairs have a non-skid surface? 41

Safety Assessment Question: Are there light switches at the top and bottom of staircases and/or hallways? 42

Safety Assessment Question: Is there adequate lighting for safely moving in the hallway or stairwell? 42

Safety Assessment Question: Is there clutter or obstacles on the stairs? 43

Safety Assessment Question: Are there solid handrails on both sides of the stairway? 43

Safety Assessment Question: Are there grade changes at entrances or between flooring changes that could be a trip hazard? 44

Safety Assessment Question: Does the elder wear anti-slip footwear? 45

Safety Assessment Question: Does the elder remove their reading glasses when using the stairs? 45

Chapter Five: Home Safety – Kitchen 47

Safety Assessment Question: Does the refrigerator contain outdated or expired food items? 47

Safety Assessment Question: Food safety: Do food items have proper storage, expiry dates? 47

Safety Assessment Question: Is a thermometer present and is the fridge within a safe operating temperature? 47

Safety Assessment Question: Are commonly used items stored towards the front of the fridge? 48

Safety Assessment Question: Is there a stable step stool (with a safety rail) for reaching high places? 49

Safety Assessment Question: Is food easy for the elder to find without using stools or ladders? 49

Safety Assessment Question: Is the elder able to buy groceries independently? & does the elder keep a well-stocked pantry and a variety of fresh fruit and vegetables on hand? 49

Safety Assessment Question: Are heavy items stored in the lower cupboards and light items in the higher cupboards? 50

Safety Assessment Question: Are all the items regularly used in the kitchen within reach? ... 50

Safety Assessment Question: Do items need to be carried a distance to the kitchen? 51

Safety Assessment Question: Are pots and pans, canned goods and staple foods stored in an easy–to–reach location--between knee and shoulder heights? 51

Safety Assessment Question: Are spills wiped up immediately? 51

Cooking: 51

Safety Assessment Question: Are there automatic devices to turn off the stove & oven? 52

Safety Assessment Question: Does the elder point pot handles away from the edge of the stove when cooking? 52

Safety Assessment Question: Are the stove knobs/dials accessible to the elder? 52

Safety Assessment Question: Are kitchen counters easy for the elder to reach? 53

Safety Assessment Question: Are oven mitts within easy reach when the elder is cooking? .. 53

Safety Assessment Question: Are knives stored safely? 53

Safety Assessment Question: Are kitchen work areas adequately illuminated? 54

Safety Assessment Question: Are appliance cords in good condition? 54

Safety Assessment Question: Are hazardous items stored separately from food? 54

Safety Assessment Question: Are the "off" and "on" positions on the stove dials clearly marked? 55

Safety Assessment Question: Are there scatter mats or throw rugs in use in the kitchen? 55

Safety Assessment Question: Are faucets easy to turn on and off? 55

Safety Assessment Question: Does the elder use the stove or oven for supplementary heat? 56

Safety Assessment Question: Does the elder use a grease splash guard when cooking greasy foods? 56

Safety Assessment Question: Is the hot water temperature set to prevent scalds? 57

Safety Assessment Question: Are smoke & carbon monoxide detectors in place and with charged batteries? 57

Safety Assessment Question: Does the elder have a cordless phone within easy reach? 57

Safety Assessment Question: Are power cords or power bars in use? Are they overloaded?. 58

Safety Assessment Question: Do you have a fire extinguisher in the kitchen, mounted on the wall away from the stove? 58

Safety Assessment Question: Are emergency numbers posted e.g. Poison Control, family members? 58

Safety Assessment Question: Does the elder use a walking aid? 59

Safety Assessment Question: Is the elder aware of foods that may interact adversely with their medications? 59

Safety Devices for the kitchen: 60

Chapter Six: Home Safety – Bathrooms 61

Safety Assessment Question: Is the bathroom clean and tidy? 61

Safety Assessment Question: Are all electrical outlets in the bathroom GFCIs? Are they tested regularly? 61

Safety Assessment Question: If incontinence products are being used, are the used supplies being disposed of properly? 62

Safety Assessment Question: Does the elder's bathroom door lock have an emergency release so it can be unlocked from both sides? 62

Safety Assessment Question: Does the elder use a walking aid? 62

Fall & Slipping Prevention: 63

Safety Assessment Question: Do bathmats next to the tub or shower have rubberized backing to prevent the elder from slipping? 63

Safety Assessment Question: Are grab bars present, properly placed and well anchored to the wall beside the bathtub or in the shower? 63

Safety Assessment Question: If an elder prefers or is required to use a shower, are grab bars and a nonslip flooring in place? 64

Safety Assessment Question: Does the bathtub have a skid proof bottom? Are grab rails available? is there a bathmat with a non-slip bottom? 64

Safety Assessment Question: Are there any trip hazards in the bathroom e.g. loose mats? .. 65

Safety Assessment Question: If it's difficult for the elder to take a shower standing up, have they considered a bath seat? 65

Safety Assessment Question: Does the elder fear getting in and/or out of the bathtub? 65

Safety Assessment Question: Are cold and hot faucets clearly marked? 66

Safety Assessment Question: Is the hot water temperature set to the recommended 49°C (120°F) to prevent scalding? 66

Safety Assessment Question: Does the elder test the water temperature before they get into the bathtub or shower? 66

Safety Assessment Question: Is the elder able to use the toilet independently and safely? ... 67

Safety Assessment Question: Are cold and hot faucets clearly marked? 67

Safety Assessment Question: Is there a night light in the bathroom? 67

Safety Assessment Question: If medication is stored in the bathroom, is it safe & secure? ... 68

Safety Assessment Question: Do bathroom cleaning products in use create slipperiness? 68

Safety Assessment Question: Are bathroom cleaning products harsh or caustic? 68

Safety Assessment Question: Is mildew present in the bathroom? 69

Safety Assessment Question: Is the elder able to use the telephone? Is telephone accessible in an emergency? 69

Safety Measures for the Bathroom: 70

Daily activities of the elder that may increase risk: 70

Chapter Seven: Home Safety – Bedrooms 71

Safety Assessment Question: Is there a clear path from the elder's bed to the bathroom? ... 71

Safety Assessment Question: Is there a phone and a list of emergency phone numbers near the elder's bed? 71

Safety Assessment Question: Are there night lights or other sources of light on in case the elder gets up in the middle of the night? 72

Safety Assessment Question: Is there a lamp or a light switch near the elder's bed? 72

Safety Assessment Question: Is there a light switch near the entrance to the elder's bedroom? 73

Safety Measures: 73

Safety Assessment Question: Is the bed height easy for the elder to get in and out of bed?.. 73

Safety Assessment Question: Assess whether door locks are required on bedroom doors to keep the elder out of other rooms or to prevent them from being locked in theirs................ 73

Safety Devices: 74

Chapter Eight: Home Safety - The Great Outdoors 75

Safety Assessment Question: Do the doorways to your balcony or deck have a low sill or threshold? 75

Safety Assessment Question: Are there solid handrails on both sides of an outdoor stairway? 75

Safety Assessment Question: Do outdoor steps and thresholds cause a hazard for elderly residents? 76

Safety Assessment Question: Are there stairs outside of the home the elder must navigate to enter/exit the home? 76

Safety Assessment Question: Look at access to decks and porch areas. Is there a step to the patio? Is there a sliding door threshold to step over? 77

Safety Assessment Question: Can the elder reach their mailbox safely and easily? 77

Safety Assessment Question: Is the number of the house clearly visible from the street and well-lit at night? 77

Neighborhood Risks: 78

Safety Assessment Question: Are there any risks inherent to the neighborhood of the elder's home? 78

Remain safe in the home: 78

Safety Assessment Question: Is the home safe for a professional caregiver to visit the home? 79

Safety Assessment Question: Is there patio furniture that would cause problems for an elder to get in and out of? 79

Safety Assessment Question: Are there any damaged steps or cracks in outdoor sidewalks? 80

Safety Assessment Question: Are there any hazards such as leaves and ice on outside pathways? 80

Safety Assessment Question: Does the elder use a motorized scooter? 81

Safety Assessment Question: Are emergency plans in place such as leaving a key with a neighbor in the case of the elder being locked out? 81

Safety Assessment Question: Are BBQ grills locked & covered when not in use? 81

Safety Assessment Question: If you live in an area that has seasonal snow falls, are there plans in place for timely snow removal? 82

Miscellaneous Outdoor Safety Devices: 82

Safety Assessment Question: Does the elder smoke outside? 84

Home Use Medical Devices 85

Chapter Nine: Electrical Safety 87

Safety Assessment Question: Is there good lighting in stairways & hallways? 88

Safety Assessment Question: Does every room have proper lighting, including walk-in closets? 88

Safety Assessment Question: Is there a lamp or a light switch near the elder's bed? 88

Safety Assessment Question: Are there light switches at the top and bottom of your staircases and/or hallways? 89

Safety Assessment Question: Is there adequate lighting for safely moving in the hallway or stairwell? 89

Safety Assessment Question: Are there night lights or other sources of light in case the elder gets up in the middle of the night? 89

Safety Assessment Questions: Is there a light switch near the entrance to the elder's bedroom? & Is there a night light in the bathroom? 90

Safety Assessment Question: Are controls & switches reachable from a wheelchair or bed? 90

Electrical Outlets, Power Bars & Extension Cords 91

Safety Assessment Question: Are electrical outlets or power bars overloaded or used unsafely e.g. daisy-chained? 91

Safety Assessment Question: Are electrical cords or cables exposed in a way that could be a trip hazard? 91

Safety Assessment Question: Are appliance cords in good condition? 92

Electrical Safety Devices for the kitchen: 92

Safety Assessment Question: Is an automatic stove shut off device in place? 92

Electrical Safety Devices for the Bathroom: 93

Safety Assessment Questions: Are all electrical outlets in the bathroom GFCIs and are they tested regularly? 93

Home Heating: 93

Safety Assessment Question: Does the home have an adequate heating system or does the elder use the stove or oven to provide heat? 93

Safety Assessment Question: If the elder uses a space heater, is it placed well away from flammable substances and materials? 94

Chapter Ten: Fire Safety & Prevention 95

Safety Assessment Question: Have you developed an escape route in case of fire and a fire safety plan?... 95

Safety Assessment Question: If the elder uses a portable space heater, is it placed well away from flammable substances and materials? 96

Safety Assessment Question: If the elder uses a portable space heater, is it plugged into the wall or to an extension cord/power bar? 96

Prevent Poisoning: Carbon Monoxide.. 98

Safety Assessment Question: If the home is older, have you or an electrician inspected the house wiring, fuse box, electrical cords and appliances for safety? 98

Safety Assessment Question: If the elder cooks, do they practice safe cooking techniques? . 99

Safety Assessment Question: Does your elder smoke? 99

Safety Assessment Question: Does the elder drink alcohol? 100

Safety Assessment Question: Are flammable and hazardous materials clearly labeled and properly stored? Is there a designated danger zone in the home to store hazardous chemicals or products?... 100

General Fire Prevention Safety Measures.. 101

Chapter Eleven: Ongoing Follow-up 103

CONCLUSION 105

CONNECT WITH US... 107

ABOUT THE AUTHOR.. 108

ALSO BY RAE A. STONEHOUSE 109

Introduction

It is often said "it takes a village to raise a child."

The same can be said about helping an elder age at home.

Perhaps not a village, but certainly a family.

With advancements in modern medicine, our aging population, on the whole, is living longer.

While many elders are living longer, they are not necessarily living better. Many are living with complex chronic medical conditions, requiring ongoing monitoring and support.

Those who would have succumbed to acute or chronic diseases and ailments in the past are continuing to live longer lives due to the benefits of ongoing medication.

We can't generalize or lump all seniors or elderly people into a one-size-fits-all category. Many seniors remain active, vibrant and mentally alert into their 90s. Yet, others seem old in their early 60s.

Caregiving at home has proven its value in offsetting the high costs of in-facility healthcare, and at the same time, improving the quality of life for many elders. However, educational training and support for caregivers has been in short supply.

Traditionally, in many cultures, the role of caring for and supporting aging parents has fallen to an unmarried daughter.

The caregiving role has changed over the years with many men stepping into the role. There is a current trend of younger people in their late teens and early 20s taking on the caretaking role for their parents who may be aging or suffering from chronic illnesses.

Taking on the role of supporting an elder living independently in the community or living with your family in your home can be an immense and daunting responsibility.

Our formal education and training haven't prepared us to take on the role of caregiver. So how do we do it?

This book is a companion workbook to the main book, **Make it Safe! A Family Caregivers Home Safety Assessment Guide for Supporting Elders@Home.** It can be purchased on-line at https://makeitsafe.online for an immediate download of an e-book. A paperback version can also be ordered on the same page.

The focus of this book is to help you as a family caregiver create a safe living space and conditions to support an elder living semi-independently in the community or adapting your family household to support an elder as a member of your family.

Make it Safe! A Family Caregivers Home Safety Guide for Supporting Elders@Home started as a module focusing on elderly safety in the Elder@Home Awareness Program which I had been contracted as a consultant to create and facilitate for a local non-profit organization.

This workbook focuses on the safety inspection portion of the main book and is designed for you to take with you when you do your assessment. Spaces are included for you to write your notes or comments in the book.

After our introduction of home safety concerns, we move on to an overview of general home safety matters. We systematically work our way through the home, focusing on specific rooms or areas where we are provided with **Safety Assessment Questions** to answer.

Many of the safety assessment questions are accompanied by **Considerations** to help you decide your course of action as well as the **Rationale** behind the question. That is, why is it important and why do you need to care about this potential problem. Each question is backed up with **Action Items** to suggest what you can or need to do to solve the problem and make it safe for you, your family and the elder.

Each hazardous item identified will also have blank lines included so you may fill in your comments, anything you want to remember or make note of completing your assessment. This workbook is meant to work for you.

Rae A. Stonehouse, Author
June 2020

Chapter One: Home Safety Overview

If you are a parent, you will probably remember what it was like to make your home safe for your children.

Many of the same principles apply when making your home safe for elders. Whereas, with children you are usually protecting them from accessing something that could be hazardous and could cause them harm, when making the home safe for elders, you will also be thinking about <u>accessibility</u>, <u>accommodating decreased mobility</u> and <u>memory deficits</u>.

At the same time, you need to be able to support the elder in maintaining their independence as long as you can and as long as they are able.

In this section we look at making your home safer for an elder to reside with you or making adaptations to the elder's current home, allowing them to live independently, with your support.

Throughout the book I use the terms 'elder', 'senior' and 'loved one' interchangeably. While this book is written from the perspective of helping an older person to live safely either independently or semi-independently in their own home, or yours, the same safety principles apply to caring for someone who is not elderly.

To do so, we will be drawing from the field of <u>personal safety</u> as a way to organize ourselves.

Introducing the 3 As of Personal safety… <u>Awareness, Assessment and Action.</u>

Awareness: As we go about the activities of our daily life, we likely encounter many situations or conditions that are hazardous. Hopefully, we have learned how to avoid or prevent negative results from these hazards.

This is <u>your</u> awareness. You realize a particular situation could be hazardous to you, so you take avoidant or corrective actions to prevent harm or injury.

This section on home safety will serve to raise your awareness on how the safety needs of an elder can be greater than what we may be used to.

I would suspect upon completion of this book you will identify hazards in your home needing rectifying for the benefit of your entire family, not just an elderly person as I did when developing this program.

Assessment: At a basic level, assessment is where you will be doing a walk-about inspection of the elder's living environment.

Much the same as a home inspector would do an investigation of a home you were considering purchasing... letting you know what is right or wrong with the house, you will be conducting a safety inspection of the elder's home.

As we work our way through the book, we will be exploring a collection of safety-related questions, focusing on different areas of the home.

The chapters are organized in main areas common to most homes and suggestions are provided to the questions posed.

As you work your way through the content, you will notice there are specific hazards common to many areas of the home. They will be identified in the chapter you are reading. To draw attention to their importance, some will have their own specific chapter examples: Fire Safety and Electrical Safety.

If you can think of a safety concern we missed, please let us know so we can share with others.

Home Safety Assessment Form: I have created a set of question sheets you can print and carry with you to complete your inspection. You can download a copy of the form at
https://BookHip.com/SXGMBT

It can be helpful to use a clipboard when you are performing your safety inspection.

Action: It doesn't help anybody if you identify a hazard and don't do anything to resolve it.

Resolving a problem may mean taking a piece of equipment such as a toaster with a faulty cord out of service, repairing a hazard or perhaps undergoing a major renovation to accommodate the elder's needs.

Create a Safety Upgrade Budget.

There are several steps to creating a budget for safety upgrades.

Some fixes you may be able to do fairly quickly. Others may take time to organize and to raise the funds to pay for the upgrades.

Once you identify a safety hazard needing improving, you need to research the options available and determine a cost.

As well, are you able to make the improvements yourself, or will you require a professional tradesperson to make the improvements? This will affect the costs involved in the home improvement.

While we complete our safety inspection, we will keep track of items that may require a budget to rectify.

Depending on where you live, there may be government or NGO (non-government organizations) funds you could access to offset the costs of home safety improvements.

In the next chapter we start our home inspection _inside_ the home. We look in detail at specific hazards and provide commentary on further considerations.

As we work our way through our home inspection, we also look at safety devices that can be purchased to solve safety problems or to facilitate the elder's continued level of functioning.

Please note we are not recommending specific products and you should undertake your due diligence before purchasing any product and putting it into service.

This page has been intentionally left blank.

Chapter Two: Home Safety - Indoors General

In this chapter we look at general areas of safety concern within the home. We expand upon many of them in upcoming chapters.

>Action: Do a walk about assessment

Take the **Home Safety Assessment Form** with you and do a walk about inspection of the inside of the elder's home.

If the elder lives with you, you could very well be conducting an assessment of your own home, however with a different set of eyes I.e. with the safety of an elder in mind.

This section of the book is organized by offering you a series of **Safety Assessment Questions.**

We follow along with the **3 A's of Personal Safety** formula discussed in the previous chapter.

Many of the questions present you with the **Rationale** behind the question i.e. the logic or reason behind the assessment question.

Some questions will also offer you **Considerations** to help you make your decision as to determining your next step.

Finally, **Action Items** will be provided to guide you to possible solutions for the hazards you have identified.

If you see a safety hazard, make it safe as soon as possible.

If you see a safety hazard, fix it as soon as possible. It may be a simple fix of taking a defective appliance out of service. Other fixes may take time and/or need to be budgeted for.

As you work your way through the home inspection, make note of items you will need to follow-up on resolving or investigating further.

There are a lot of items in this inspection and it can be easy to want to start solving problems before you complete your assessment.

Stay the course. Complete your home assessment, then create your action plan to resolve items identified. Perhaps solving the easy ones first might be a good start.

Safety Assessment Question: Is house clean & tidy?

Considerations: Is the home reasonably clean and tidy? Is the house stocked with dish soap, laundry soap and other cleaning supplies?

Action Item: if the home isn't tidy, make note of the fact and return to this item upon completion of your assessment. At that time make a list of areas needing tidying and create a list of cleaning supplies you may need to be purchased.

Notes:_____
_____
_____
_____
_____
_____

Safety Assessment Question: Is the home safe for a professional caregiver to visit the home?

Rationale: Professional caregivers are trained to consider their own health and safety first. If the home presents a potential hazard to their personal safety, they may deny service until the hazard has been rectified.

If the elder is a smoker, they may be required to refrain from smoking for a specific amount of time to reduce the hazards of second-hand smoke to the caregiver.

Action Item: if the elder requires the services of a professional caregiver who provides services within the elder's home, speak to the caregiver about their requirements and/or health & safety needs.

Notes:_____
_____
_____
_____
_____
_____

Safety Assessment Question: Are emergency numbers posted?

Considerations: Emergency numbers include: poison control, physicians, most responsible family member, 911 for police, fire or ambulance, an involved neighbor, etc.

Action Items:
a) If an Emergency Number List hasn't been created, make one.

b) Post the list in an easily accessible location such as the refrigerator.

Notes:_____
_____
_____
_____
_____
_____

Safety Assessment Question: Is there a designated danger zone in the home to store hazardous chemicals or products?

Rationale: People with dementia forget the purpose of things and how to use them. They may think wiper fluid is juice or be unaware that the grill is hot.

Action Items:
a. Designate a danger zone.

b. To make the home safer, turn the garage, workroom, closet, outdoor shed, recycled TV armoire or a large cabinet into a storage place for:
- cleaning products
- bleach
- mothballs
- insecticide
- paint, turpentine, stain
- sharp knives, scissors, box cutters, blades
- alcohol
- tobacco products, including chewing tobacco
- hand and power tools

Better still, remove these products completely from the home and find alternative storage. You could then bring them with you when you visited the home if you required them.

  c. Install key or combination locks on rooms and other storage places containing potentially dangerous items. In addition, use childproof doorknob covers or cabinet locks.

Notes:_____
_____
_____
_____
_____
_____

Safety Assessment Question: Is there good lighting in stairways & hallways?

  Considerations: Make home lighting brighter but prevent glare.

  Action Item: Provide good lighting where required.

Notes:_____
_____
_____
_____
_____
_____

Safety Assessment Question: Does every room have proper lighting, including walk-in closets?

  Action Items:
  a. Ensure every room has proper lighting, including walk-in closets. Use a nightlight to make it easy to see at night. Battery operated nightlights are available for areas without electrical access.

  b. Place a light (such as a lamp) close to the bed and make sure the elder can reach it easily.

  c. Extra lamps: consider models that turn on and off with a touch.

Notes:_____
_____
_____

Safety Assessment Question: Are light switches installed at the top and bottom of staircases?

    Action Item: If not present, install light switches at the top and bottom of your staircases.

Notes:_____
_____
_____
_____
_____
_____

Safety Assessment Question: Are bookshelves anchored to walls to prevent toppling over?

    Action Item: Ensure bookshelves are anchored to walls. Heavy duty anti-tip furniture straps are readily available for purchase at your local hardware store.

Notes:_____
_____
_____
_____
_____
_____

Safety Assessment Questions: Is a smoke and carbon monoxide detector present?
Do the detectors work?
When were the batteries last changed?
How often are the batteries changed and by whom?

    Rationale: Carbon monoxide is a deadly, odorless, colorless gas—you cannot smell it or see it. Having a working carbon monoxide detector is crucial to elder safety! And to your own...

    Action Item: If your smoke or carbon monoxide detectors are more than 10 years old, it's time to replace them!

Notes:_____
_____
_____

_____
_____
_____

Safety Assessment Question: Are there any wheeled swivel chairs in the home?

    Rationale: Wheeled swivel chairs can be a danger to an elderly person. The chair can easily move out from under them when they attempt to sit or get up from.

    Action Item: If practical, remove the wheels from the chair.
Or remove from the home or keep in a room the elder doesn't have access to.

Notes:_____
_____
_____
_____
_____
_____
_____

Safety Assessment Question: Do bedrooms or bathrooms have locks that can be released should an elder lock themselves in?

    Rationale: Cabinet locks, door guardians, and refrigerator locks can prevent access to storage areas or exits from the house to discourage wandering or exploring, which might end badly.

    Action Items:
        a.   Remove locks from bedroom and bathroom doors so you can get in quickly, should the elder fall.

        b.   Switch out standard doorknobs for lever handles.

Notes:_____
_____
_____
_____
_____
_____

Safety Assessment Question: Are doorways and halls wide enough for an elder to navigate with a wheelchair or walker?

Action Item: If required: offset door hinges to make room for a wheelchair, walker or two people walking side by side.

Notes:_____
_____
_____
_____
_____
_____

Safety Assessment Question: Are cordless phones within easy reach of the elder?

Action Item: Have a cordless phone at the elder's home and keep it within easy reach, to prevent having to rush to answer when the phone rings.

Consideration: If you are purchasing new cordless phones, consider a multi-unit set. This will allow you to have one unit in the charger which you can easily swap out with one with a reduced power charge whenever you visit the elder's home.

Notes:_____
_____
_____
_____
_____
_____

Safety Assessment Questions: Is the furniture stable?

Do chairs wobble when sat in?

Are chair arms, seat cushions, chair backs, etc. all in good condition?

Action Items:
a. Ensure all furniture an elder might use in their daily activity is safe for use. If not, either repair the item or remove from service.

b. Discard or donate old furniture.

Notes:_____
_____
_____
_____
_____
_____

Safety Assessment Question: Are furniture cushion levels at the right level to allow the elder to easily sit down?

Action Item: Use firm foam cushions to raise the height of furniture.

Notes:_____
_____
_____
_____
_____
_____

Safety Assessment Question: Are electrical cords or cables exposed in a way that could be a trip hazard?

Action Item: Avoid stretching extension cords across the floor.

Notes:_____
_____
_____
_____
_____
_____

Safety Assessment Question: Are there any barriers to creating a safe home?

Notes:_____
_____
_____
_____

Safety Assessment Question: Are bed rails required for the elder sleeping safety?

    Consideration: If already in place, are they being used safely & correctly?

Notes:_____
_____
_____
_____
_____
_____

Safety Assessment Question: Is the elder's bed at a level that allows them to place their feet on the floor when attempting to stand up from the bed?

    Consideration: Pay attention to the height of the elder's bed: if their feet can't touch the floor while sitting on the bed, it means their bed is too high.

    Action Items:
        a.   Try lowering the bed by removing their box spring.

        b.   Similarly, if their knees are higher than their hips while sitting, it means the bed is too low. In this case, try adding a box spring.

Notes:_____
_____
_____
_____
_____
_____

Safety Assessment Question: Is the elder's clothing safe?

    Consideration: Does the elder wear clothing that may become a hazard?

    Examples: Loose sleeves can become entangled in appliances or a fire hazard when cooking on the stove, ties can become caught in household appliances.

    Action Items: Observe the clothing the elder wears when cooking. If the sleeves or other aspect of the clothing appears to be hazardous, suggest to the elder to change their clothing to something safer.

Notes:_____
_____
_____
_____
_____
_____

Safety Assessment Question: Does the home have an adequate heating system or does the elder use the stove or oven to provide heat?

Consideration: Heat the home safely – do not use an oven as a heating source, under any circumstance.

Action Item: Encourage the elder to turn off all portable heaters if and when they leave the home.

Notes:_____
_____
_____
_____
_____
_____

Safety Assessment Question: Have you developed an escape route in case of fire and a fire safety plan?

Action Item: We discuss this in detail in an upcoming chapter on fire safety.

Notes:_____
_____
_____
_____
_____
_____

Safety Assessment Question: If the elder uses a space heater, is it placed well away from flammable substances and materials?

Action Item: We also discuss this in detail in an upcoming chapter on fire safety.

Notes:_____
_____
_____
_____
_____
_____

Safety Assessment Question: Is there any evidence of leaks in the home as evidenced by water stains on a ceiling or an interior wall?

Rationale: Water stains on a ceiling or actively dripping water can indicate a leaky roof or perhaps a problem with a leaky toilet, bathtub or shower.

Action Items:
- a. Check for leaks in the roof around windows and doors.
- b. Replace broken windows, which can allow for cold air to enter the room.
- c. If water leakage and damage is due to a plumbing leak, have a qualified plumber solve the problem.

Safety Assessment Question: Do you have a first aid kit and know where it is?

Action Item: Is the first aid kit checked regularly to ensure supplies are replenished?

Miscellaneous Safety Measures:

In the next part of this chapter we look at a collection of miscellaneous safety measures to help an elder live safely in our home or in their own home.

Cover furniture corners to prevent injuries if you accidentally bump into them.

Water Heater Temperature:

Rationale: As we age, our skin and body fat can become thinner. This can cause an elder to bruise and burn easier than a younger person.

Action Item: If you have a water boiler/hot water heater, don't set the thermostat to "Hot". Instead, use the "Medium" setting to avoid burns or scalding.

Notes:_____
_____
_____
_____
_____
_____

Mixing cleaning products:

Do not mix cleaning products together—some substances may be extremely dangerous when combined.

    Rationale: For example, one of the most common hazards occurs when chlorine bleach is mixed with ammonia or acids.

    The combination of ammonia and bleach produces dangerous chlorine gas, which in small doses can cause irritation to the eyes, skin and respiratory tract.

    In large doses, it can kill. Chlorine gas, also known as mustard gas, was actually used in WWI & WWII.

Controls & switches that are reachable from a wheelchair or bed:

    Action Item: If possible, are you able to relocate controls and switches so they are reachable from a wheelchair or bed?

Notes:_____
_____
_____
_____
_____
_____

Laundry facilities on first floor:

    Rationale: Many older homes have a laundry area set up in the basement. Having to go up and down the basement steps repeatedly can be troublesome for an elder with mobility problems.

    There can also be other safety concerns inherent with a basement laundry room such as inadequate lighting, dampness/wetness, flooring surface hazards.

Action Item: If practical, move laundry facilities to the first floor.

Notes:_____
_____
_____
_____
_____
_____

Is the furniture I.e. living room chairs and couches, kitchen chairs, etc. Easy for the elder to get in and out of?

Rationale: The elder may have difficulty getting in and out of low furniture.

Action Item: Remove small and low furniture.

Large Screen Televisions:

Rationale: With larger screen televisions becoming commonplace, a hazard can be created for an elder who may be unsteady on their feet. A trip or a stumble can cause an unsecured television to fall, creating an electrical and/or glass breakage hazard.

Action Item: Stabilize unsecured large screen televisions to the wall with a security strap. These can be purchased at electronics or hardware stores.

Notes:_____
_____
_____
_____
_____
_____

Safety Devices:

Use a Reacher device.

Rationale: Reacher devices are an inexpensive and effective tool for extending the reach of an elder. Yours too for that matter.

Be sure to not lift anything breakable or too heavy when using a Reacher device.

Action Item: Obtain a Reacher device and demonstrate to the elder how to use it.

Notes:_____
_____
_____
_____
_____
_____

Floor to ceiling pole:

Rationale: Many elderly have mobility problems making getting in and out of their bed or bathtub, or perhaps their favorite chair, quite difficult for them to manage

There are several inexpensive models of ceiling poles on the market that can be easily installed. Multiple poles can be purchased and installed in key areas such as the elder's bedroom, their bathroom and the living room.

Action Items:
a. Install a floor to ceiling pole or other assistive devices for the person to hold on to when rising from furniture.

b. You should demonstrate to the elder how to use the equipment safely and effectively. They should also be monitored to ensure they follow through with using it appropriately.

Notes:_____
_____
_____
_____
_____
_____
_____

Hip pads:

Action Item: Encourage the elder to wear hip pads should they be at risk for falls.

Notes:_____
_____
_____
_____

Seating at the Home Entrance:

Make it Safe TIP: Install a seat at the entrance of your home to remove or put on your shoes and boots.

Notes:_____
_____
_____
_____
_____
_____

Safety Suggestions

Go slow up and down stairs.

Rationale: Don't rush going up or down stairs. Rushing is a major cause of falls.

Eye glasses and climbing stairs:

Does the elder remove their reading glasses when using the stairs?

Notes:_____
_____
_____
_____
_____
_____

Keep it Safe TIP: Car keys should be inaccessible. This assumes of course that the elder is no longer driving and/or may be confused.

Firearms should be kept in a gun safe or off the property.

Notes:_____
_____
_____

∽

In the next chapter we focus on assessing fall hazards in the elder's home.

This page has been intentionally left blank.

Chapter Three: Assessing Fall Hazards

In this chapter we look at potential fall hazards within the elder's home and offer solutions to prevent them.

Remove Fall Hazards.

To reduce the risk of falls for seniors, one of the most important actions you can take is to make the home fall-safe.

Safety Assessment Question: Do the steps of the stairs have a non-skid surface?

Action Item: Install nonskid treads on steps if not present.

Note: We discuss steps and stairs in depth in upcoming chapters.

Notes:_____
_____
_____
_____
_____
_____

Safety Assessment Question: Are there solid handrails on both sides of the stairway?

Action Item: If handrails are not present, install a handrail on at least one side of the stairway.

Notes:_____
_____
_____
_____
_____
_____

Safety Assessment Question: Are pets underfoot?

Action Item: This isn't an easy question to supply an action for. Many pets are clingy and tend to stay very close to their owners. If the elder requires the in-house services of a healthcare professional, it might be a good idea to secure the pet in another closed room for the duration of the visit.

Notes:_____
_____
_____
_____
_____
_____

Safety Assessment Question: Are household pathways clear?

    Considerations: Consider developing storage or organization systems to help deal with the clutter.

    Action Items:
        a.   Ensure household pathways are clear.

        b.   Remove clutter.

Notes:_____
_____
_____
_____
_____
_____

Safety Assessment Question: Does the elder wear anti-slip footwear within the house?

    Action Items: Encourage the elder to wear supportive, ant-slip footwear within the house as well as when outdoors.

Notes:_____
_____
_____
_____
_____
_____

Safety Assessment Question: Are there grade changes at entrances or between flooring changes?

Action Item: Adjust grade changes at entrances or between flooring changes.

Notes:_____
_____
_____
_____
_____
_____

Safety Assessment Question: Do door sills present a potential tripping hazard?

Action Items:

    a.   If possible, adjust threshold entryways to remove a difference in elevations between rooms.

    b.   Paint door sills with a different highlighting color to help avoid tripping.

Notes:_____
_____
_____
_____
_____
_____

Safety Assessment Question: Is there any clutter on the stairs?

Action Item: Ensure there is no clutter or obstacles on the stairs. Clean up loose clutter. This includes newspapers, loose clothing and shoes.

Notes:_____
_____
_____
_____
_____
_____

Safety Assessment Question: Is the elder able to climb and descend stairs easily or with difficulty?

Action Item: If stairs are too difficult for older adults to safely use, consider installing a stair glide or having the elder stay on the main level.

Notes:_____
_____
_____
_____
_____
_____

Safety Assessment Question: Are there any small furniture items that could be a trip hazard?

Action Items:

    a.   To prevent fall risks, use cord covers for all cords and cables, or secure them out of the way, behind furniture.

    b.   If carpet is loose or wrinkled, or the floors are damaged or uneven, have them repaired.

    c.   Remove foot stools and small tables from the living room if not essential to the elder's functioning.

Notes:_____
_____
_____
_____
_____
_____

Safety Assessment Question: Are the home's high-traffic areas clear of obstacles?

Action Item: As you walk through the home, consider how it would be for an elder to navigate with a cane, a walker or a wheelchair.

Considerations: If obstacles to navigation are identified, is it possible to remove the obstacle or change it so that it doesn't provide a hazard?

Notes:_____
_____
_____
_____
_____
_____

Safety Assessment Question: If you use floor wax, do you use the non-skid kind?

Action Item: If floor wax is required, switch to the non-skid type.

Notes:_____
_____
_____
_____
_____
_____
_____

∼

In the next chapter we look at safety hazards in specific areas of the home, starting with hallways and stairwells.

This page has been intentionally left blank.

Chapter Four: Home Safety - Hallways & Stairwells

Safety Assessment:

Action: Do a walk around safety assessment.

Take the **Home Safety Assessment Form** with you and do a walk about inspection of the hallways and stairwells of the elder's home.

As mentioned earlier, there may be some duplication of the possible hazards identified and solutions offered.

Notes:_____
_____
_____
_____
_____
_____
_____

Safety Assessment Question: Are household pathways clear?

Considerations: Consider developing storage or organization systems to help deal with the clutter.

Action Items:
    a.   Ensure household pathways are clear.

    b.   Remove clutter.

Notes:_____
_____
_____
_____
_____
_____
_____

Safety Assessment Question: Do the steps of your stairs have a non-skid surface?

Action Items:
    a.   If stairs are difficult for older adults to safely use, consider installing a stair glide or having the elder stay on the main level.

b. Install rubber stair treads to provide grip to an otherwise slippery set of stairs.

Notes:_____
_____
_____
_____
_____
_____

Safety Assessment Question: Are there light switches at the top and bottom of staircases and/or hallways?

Rationale: Older homes may only have a light switch installed at the bottom of the staircase or one end of the hallway. This would necessitate you having to go back to the source to turn it off again, which could create risk walking in the dark.

Action Item: Install light switches at the top and bottom of your staircases. This installation would require the services of a qualified electrician.

Notes:_____
_____
_____
_____
_____
_____

Safety Assessment Question: Is there adequate lighting for safely moving in the hallway or stairwell?

Rationale: The existing light fixtures may be adequate if a suitable light bulb is installed. There are a variety of lightbulbs available e.g. halogen and LED that provide more light, last longer, shed less heat and are more economical to operate.

Action Item: Ensure there is good lighting in stairways and hallways.

Consideration: If good lighting is not present e.g. inappropriately placed, it may be necessary to contact a qualified electrician to install additional fixtures.

Notes:_____
_____
_____
_____
_____
_____

Safety Assessment Question: Is there clutter or obstacles on the stairs?

Rationale: Clothing, books, etc. can easily pile up at the top and bottom of the stairs waiting for someone to carry them up or down at the next opportunity.

With many elderly experiencing visual challenges, these piles of clutter can easily become a trip hazard for them or anyone else for that matter.

Action Item: Ensure there is no clutter or obstacles on the stairs.

Considerations: Some people find it helpful to keep a laundry basket near the stairs, but not so it creates a hazard, to store items to be taken to the next level when enough of a load is gathered.

Notes:_____
_____
_____
_____
_____
_____

Safety Assessment Question: Are there solid handrails on both sides of the stairway?

Rationale: You don't need to be a home handyman to do this. Grab the railing and try to shake it back and forth. If the railing wiggles (even somewhat), it's time to fix it. Tighten all nuts and bolts or replace the railing.

Action Items:
    a.   If stair railings are present, test them for stability.

    b.   If solid handrails are not present in stairways, install them on both sides of the stairs. If you are handy or have access to a handyperson, this is relatively easily done.

Considerations: It's essential the railing holders are securely fastened to the wall's studs. The railings should not cause more of a hazard than they are attempting to solve. An example might be where the rails protrude into the passageway, making it too narrow to navigate safely.

Notes:_____
_____
_____
_____
_____
_____

Safety Assessment Question: Is it easy to differentiate one step from another?

Rationale: With partial vision, an elder may be unable to separate one step from the next. This could increase the chance of the elder falling or slipping.

Action Items:

a. Differentiate between stair steps. To increase home safety for seniors, you could paint stair tops a contrasting color.

b. Stretching a piece of different-colored duct tape over the top of each stair can also make each step easier to spot. Ensure the tape doesn't become loose and create its own safety hazard.

Notes:_____
_____
_____
_____
_____
_____

Safety Assessment Question: Are there grade changes at entrances or between flooring changes that could be a trip hazard?

Rationale: Many elders have visual difficulties which can include depth perception or the inability to differentiate between two surfaces.

Considerations: Wood or metal thresholds are available at building centers. They can be cut to length and can come in various widths to accommodate the grade difference between two areas of the house.

Action Items:

a. Adjust grade changes at entrances or between flooring changes.

b. Paint door sills with a different highlighting color, by serving as a visual cue, can help avoid tripping.

Notes:_____
_____
_____
_____
_____
_____
_____

Safety Assessment Question: Does the elder wear anti-slip footwear?

Rationale: Many floor surfaces can be slippery for an elder to walk on. It is often compounded by the elder wearing footwear that might be deemed comfortable rather than safe and practical.

Action Item: Encourage the elder to wear anti-slip slippers or anti-slip socks when walking around your home, especially on slippery surfaces such as polished hardwood floors or tile.

Pool or bathing shoes may be an option for the elder when getting in and out of a bathtub.

Notes:_____
_____
_____
_____
_____
_____
_____

Safety Assessment Question: Does the elder remove their reading glasses when using the stairs?

Rationale: Reading glasses are designed for seeing close-up. Wearing them while walking up or down stairs may not provide adequate vision to navigate the stairs or to identify hazards.

Action Items:

    a. Encourage the elder to remove their reading glasses before navigating stairs.

    b. Encourage them not rush going up or down stairs. Rushing is a major cause of falls.

Considerations: Rushing to answer a telephone can be a cause of falls in the elderly.

Action Item: Provide a portable, cordless phone on each floor of the elder's home to reduce the need to rush to answer a phone.

Notes:_____
_____
_____
_____
_____
_____

In the next chapter we look at potential safety hazards in the kitchen.

Chapter Five: Home Safety – Kitchen

The kitchen is often the heart of a home. Therefore, it seems only fitting that you should spend considerable time making this room safe for an elder.

Do a walk around safety assessment.

Take the **Home Safety Assessment Form** with you and do a walk about inspection of the kitchen of the elder's home.

Go on pantry patrol.

Safety Assessment Question: Does the refrigerator contain outdated or expired food items?

Safety Assessment Question: Food safety: Do food items have proper storage, expiry dates?

Action Item: Check for proper storage of foods. Example: food products requiring refrigeration after the product is opened.

Rationale: You probably won't have any problems if foods not requiring refrigeration are placed in the fridge. However, products such as dairy products that aren't refrigerated would likely be spoiled and should be disposed.

Action Item: Check products for expiry dates and/or best before dates.

Notes:_____
_____
_____
_____
_____
_____

Safety Assessment Question: Is a thermometer present and is the fridge within a safe operating temperature?

Rationale: People with dementia may eat spoiled, expired, raw and moldy food.

Action Item: Make regular pantry and refrigerator inspections. Discard any stored foods past their "best before" date.

If necessary, adjust the refrigerator's temperature to ensure it is in the safe operating range.

Make it Safe TIP: [From Mr. Google...] The U.S. Food and Drug Administration (FDA) says the recommended refrigerator temperature is below 40°F; the ideal freezer temp is below 0°F.

However, the ideal refrigerator temperature is actually lower: Aim to stay between 35° and 38°F (or 1.7 to 3.3°C).

Rationale: When judgment becomes impaired, a jar of maraschino cherries or instant coffee crystals may seem like a good meal.

Action Items:
    a.   Put certain foods out of sight.

    b.   This might seem odd... but limit your pet's mealtimes and remove the bowl so your loved one doesn't snack on kibble.

Notes:_____
_____
_____
_____
_____
_____

Safety Assessment Question: Are commonly used items stored towards the front of the fridge?

Action Item: Store commonly used items towards the front of the fridge.

Notes:_____
_____
_____
_____
_____
_____

Make it Safe TIP: Keep a close eye on everyday appliances or permanent fixtures that can become hazards.

Safety Assessment Question: Is there a stable step stool (with a safety rail) for reaching high places?

Action Item: If it is necessary for an elder to reach into upper cupboards, ensure a step stool with a stable base and a handrail is available. It should be within easy reach for the elder. Look for a stool no more than one or two steps in height.

Notes:_____
_____
_____
_____
_____
_____

Safety Assessment Question: Is food easy for the elder to find without using stools or ladders?

Rationale: Climbing on step stools, chairs or counters is risky for people with dementia, visual perception problems or balancing problems.

Action Item: Make food easy to find and reach.

Notes:_____
_____
_____
_____
_____
_____

Safety Assessment Question: Is the elder able to buy groceries independently? & does the elder keep a well-stocked pantry and a variety of fresh fruit and vegetables on hand?

Considerations: If the elder is independent with their grocery shopping, provide assistance where needed e.g. transporting the elder to the grocery store, carrying groceries into the house from the vehicle, helping to put groceries away in kitchen cupboards or other storage areas.

If the elder is not independent...

Action Items:
    a.   Consult with the elder to create a shopping list.

    b.   If practical, take the elder with you when grocery shopping.
Stock their pantry with healthy snacks (e.g. yogurt, granola bars, nuts, cheese and crackers, and fruit).

Notes:_____
_____
_____
_____
_____
_____

Safety Assessment Question: Are heavy items stored in the lower cupboards and light items in the higher cupboards?

    Rationale: Minimize both the need to carry items and the distance the items need to be carried.

    Action Item: Store heavy items in the lower cupboards and light items in the higher cupboards.

Notes:_____
_____
_____
_____
_____
_____

Safety Assessment Question: Are all the items regularly used in the kitchen within reach?

    Action Item: Place all items you frequently use within easy reach in the kitchen – don't place them on high shelves that are hard to access.

Notes:_____
_____
_____
_____
_____

Safety Assessment Question: Do items need to be carried a distance to the kitchen?

Action Items:
    a. If the elder is not able to buy groceries independently suggest using a grocery delivery or a meal delivery service.

    b. Minimize both the need to carry items and the distance the items need to be carried.

Notes:_____
_____
_____
_____
_____
_____

Safety Assessment Question: Are pots and pans, canned goods and staple foods stored in an easy–to–reach location--between knee and shoulder heights?

Action Item: Store pots & pans, canned goods, and staple foods in an easy–to–reach location... between knee and shoulder height to minimize reaching and lifting heavy items.

Notes:_____
_____
_____
_____
_____
_____

Safety Assessment Question: Are spills wiped up immediately?

Action Item: Ensure that spills are wiped up immediately.
Provide paper towels for clean-up.

Cooking:

Safety Assessment Question: Does the elder wear loose clothing when cooking?

Action Item: If the elder does wear loose clothing when cooking, encourage them to change to something more form-fitting as loose fabric can catch fire very quickly.

Make it Safe TIP: All fabrics will burn, but some are more combustible than others.

Notes:_____
_____
_____
_____
_____
_____

Safety Assessment Question: Are there automatic devices to turn off the stove & oven?

Action Item: Replace an older kettle with an automatic shut-off mechanism.

Notes:_____
_____
_____
_____
_____
_____

Safety Assessment Question: Does the elder point pot handles away from the edge of the stove when cooking?

Action Item: Encourage your elder to point pot handles away from the front edge of the stove. This ensures that they won't bump into them or catch the handles with their sleeve.

Notes:_____
_____
_____
_____
_____
_____

Safety Assessment Question: Are the stove knobs/dials accessible to the elder?

Action Item: If the elder has difficulty reaching stove knobs, have them use a stove knob turner. Or consider appliances with the knobs at the front of the appliance.

Notes:_____
_____
_____
_____
_____
_____

Safety Assessment Question: Are kitchen counters easy for the elder to reach?

Action Item: Check to ensure your kitchen counters are easy for the elder to reach. If they are too high, it's a good idea to lower them to a more accessible height.

Notes:_____
_____
_____
_____
_____
_____

Safety Assessment Question: Are oven mitts within easy reach when the elder is cooking?

Action Item: Ensure oven mitts are within easy reach when the elder is cooking.

Make it Safe TIP: Use heat-resistant oven mitts rather than potholders; they provide a better grip on hot containers and give you better protection against splatters and steam. If you do experience a burn, immerse in cool water (not ice or butter!).

Notes:_____
_____
_____
_____
_____
_____

Safety Assessment Question: Are knives stored safely?

Action Item: Store knives and electric appliances in a cabinet with a childproof lock.

Notes:_____
_____

Safety Assessment Question: Are kitchen work areas adequately illuminated?

    Action Item: Make home lighting brighter but prevent glare.

Notes:_____
_____
_____
_____
_____
_____

Safety Assessment Question: Are appliance cords in good condition?

    Action Item: If any appliance power cords or wires are torn or frayed, replace them immediately to decrease the risk of fire.

Notes:_____
_____
_____
_____
_____
_____

Safety Assessment Question: Are hazardous items stored separately from food?

    Action Item: Store hazardous items separate from food.

    Hazardous items examples:

- o   Household cleaning products
- o   Bleach
- o   Soaps & detergents

Notes:_____
_____
_____
_____
_____
_____

Safety Assessment Question: Are the "off" and "on" positions on the stove dials clearly marked?

Action Item: Ensure the on and off stove dials are clearly marked.

Notes:_____
_____
_____
_____
_____
_____

Safety Assessment Question: Are there scatter mats or throw rugs in use in the kitchen?

Rationale: These may be decorative but often lack a rubberized backing to better grip the floor, which can become a trip and fall hazard.

Action Items:

    a.   Remove scatter mats/throw rugs.

    b.   If carpet is loose or wrinkled or the floors are damaged or uneven, have them repaired.

Notes:_____
_____
_____
_____
_____
_____

Safety Assessment Question: Are faucets easy to turn on and off?

Action Item: Provide rubberized water faucet covers for the kitchen sink. These can be easier to grip and turn and are color-coded: red for hot and blue for cold. You should be able to find these products at a senior's supply store.

Alternatively, you could replace standard 'twist and turn' kitchen water faucet handles with 'single-lever' handles instead. Older people can find these far easier to use.

Notes:_____
_____
_____
_____
_____
_____

Safety Assessment Question: Does the elder use the stove or oven for supplementary heat?

Action Item: Heat the home safely – do not use an oven as a heating source, under any circumstance. Turn off all portable heaters when leaving the home.

Notes:_____
_____
_____
_____
_____
_____

Safety Assessment Question: Does the elder use a grease splash guard when cooking greasy foods?

Action Items:
a. Wipe off any spilled grease from the stove.

b. Use a grease splash guard when cooking bacon or other greasy foods.

c. Consider using a microwave rather than the stove.

Notes:_____
_____
_____
_____
_____
_____

Safety Assessment Question: Is the hot water temperature set to prevent scalds?

Action Item: If you have a water heater, don't set the thermostat to 'Hot'. Instead, use the 'Medium' setting to avoid burns or scalding.

Notes:_____
_____
_____
_____
_____
_____

Safety Assessment Question: Are smoke & carbon monoxide detectors in place and with charged batteries?

Rationale: Remember that carbon monoxide is a deadly, odorless, colorless gas – you cannot smell it or see it. Having a working carbon monoxide detector is crucial to elder safety!

Action Item: Keep your smoke detectors and carbon monoxide detectors up to date by checking the batteries regularly and promptly replacing expired/discharged batteries.

Note: If your smoke or carbon monoxide detectors are more than 10 years old, it's time to replace them!

Notes:_____
_____
_____
_____
_____
_____

Safety Assessment Question: Does the elder have a cordless phone within easy reach?

Action Item: Have a cordless phone at home and keep it within easy reach, to prevent having to rush to answer when the phone rings.

Notes:_____
_____
_____
_____

Safety Assessment Question: Are power cords or power bars in use? Are they overloaded?

Action Item: Do not overload power sockets or extension cords.

Notes:_____
_____
_____
_____
_____
_____

Safety Assessment Question: Do you have a fire extinguisher in the kitchen, mounted on the wall away from the stove?

Action Items:
    a.   Is the fire extinguisher regularly checked to see if it is in good operating order?

    b.   Is there a record of checking available?

Notes:_____
_____
_____
_____
_____
_____

Safety Assessment Question: Are emergency numbers posted e.g. Poison Control, family members?

Action Item: Ensure emergency numbers are posted e.g. Poison Control, family members.

Notes:_____
_____
_____
_____
_____

Safety Assessment Question: Does the elder use a walking aid?

Considerations: Does the layout of the kitchen allow for the elder to navigate safely around the Kitchen?

Action Items:
    a.   Ensure the walking aid is set for the correct height for the elder.

    b.   Remove obstacles from the kitchen to allow the elder to navigate safely with or without a walking aid.

Notes:_____
_____
_____
_____
_____
_____

Safety Assessment Question: Is the elder aware of foods that may interact adversely with their medications?

Considerations: Are others aware of possible adverse reactions? One common food to avoid when taking cardiac medications is grapefruits and/or grapefruit juice.

Closely related to food and medication interactions are allergies.

Action Items:
    a.   Research the elder's medications to determine if there are any known adverse interactions to food.

    b.   Interview your elder to learn if they have any allergies you need to be aware of.

Notes:_____
_____
_____
_____
_____
_____

Safety Devices for the kitchen:

Automatic stove shut off device:

Considerations: Consider using automatic devices to turn off the stove and oven or installing an induction cooktop -- which turns off when a pot is removed from the burner. Automatic shutoffs on small appliances are recommended.

Action Items:
    a.   Install an automatic device to turn off the stove after a set period if no movement is detected.

Notes:_____
_____
_____
_____
_____
_____

In the next chapter we assess safety hazards in the elder's bathroom.

Chapter Six: Home Safety – Bathrooms

Action Item: Take the **Home Safety Assessment Form** with you and do a walk about inspection of the bathroom the elder uses on a regular basis.

Notes:_____
_____
_____
_____
_____
_____

Safety Assessment Question: Is the bathroom clean and tidy?

Rationale: The condition of the elder's bathroom can often be used as a determination of how the elder is functioning. That is, if the bathroom is clean and tidy, odds are they are doing well in other areas of daily living. Generally, older women tend to be more concerned with cleanliness than older men are.

Notes:_____
_____
_____
_____
_____
_____

Safety Assessment Question: Are all electrical outlets in the bathroom GFCIs? Are they tested regularly?

Rationale: A ground fault circuit interrupter (GFCI) will close the circuit should a person with wet hands come in contact with the receptacle, preventing the individual from being electrocuted.

Action Item: Ensure outlets in the bathroom have a ground fault circuit interrupter (GFCI) or are protected by a GFCI circuit.

Notes:_____
_____
_____
_____

Safety Assessment Question: If incontinence products are being used, are the used supplies being disposed of properly?

Rationale: Soiled incontinence products can cause unsanitary conditions if left to accumulate.

Action Items:
    a.   Provide a disposal collection container separate from regular bathroom waste.

    b.   Dispose of soiled incontinence products as necessary.

Notes:_____
_____
_____
_____
_____
_____

Safety Assessment Question: Does the elder's bathroom door lock have an emergency release so it can be unlocked from both sides?

Action Item: Install bathroom door locks that can be easily opened from the outside should an elder accidentally lock themselves in.

Notes:_____
_____
_____
_____
_____
_____

Safety Assessment Question: Does the elder use a walking aid?

Action Items:
    a.   Ensure walking aids are of the correct height for the elder.

    b.   Ensure there is enough room for maneuverability for the elder in the bathroom. This would include allowing for walkers and wheelchairs if in use.

Notes:_____
_____
_____
_____
_____
_____

Fall & Slipping Prevention:

Safety Assessment Question: Do bathmats next to the tub or shower have rubberized backing to prevent the elder from slipping?

    Action Item: Utilize rubber backed bathmats to prevent the elder from slipping when getting in or out of the shower or bathtub.

    Considerations: Having two or three bathmats available can ensure continued slip prevention when one or more mats are being laundered.

Notes:_____
_____
_____
_____
_____
_____

Safety Assessment Question: Are grab bars present, properly placed and well anchored to the wall beside the bathtub or in the shower?

    Rationale: Many grab bars are designed to also serve as towel bars, toilet paper holders and in-shower shelves.

    Action Item: Ensure there are grab bars present for the elder for toileting and bathing i.e. shower and/or tub.

Notes:_____
_____
_____
_____
_____
_____

Safety Assessment Question: If an elder prefers or is required to use a shower, are grab bars and a nonslip flooring in place?

Rationale: Shower seats and shower rails make it much easier and safer for a senior to take a shower or bath without falling, and non-slip mats placed in the tub contribute to staying balanced.

Action Items:
- a. Ensure grab bars are available within the shower.
- b. Ensure the floor to the shower is slip proof. This can be accomplished by using a removable rubber or vinyl bathmat.
- c. There are also adhesive bath treads designed for shower stall floors that can easily be applied.

An additional option is an anti-slip coating that can be applied to bathtub bottoms and shower bases.

Anti-Slip Coatings will increase friction and reduce the likelihood of a fall. The components include either a clear coat or a color-matched coating with a semi-transparent powder added to provide a textured surface.

Notes:_____
_____
_____
_____
_____
_____

Safety Assessment Question: Does the bathtub have a skid proof bottom? Are grab rails available? is there a bathmat with a non-slip bottom?

Action Item: See Action Items in the above safety assessment question.

Notes:_____
_____
_____
_____
_____

Safety Assessment Question: Are there any trip hazards in the bathroom e.g. loose mats?

Action Item: Remove any trip hazards. Examples: throw rugs, stools, etc.
Minimize clutter.

Notes:_____
_____
_____
_____
_____
_____

Safety Assessment Question: If it's difficult for the elder to take a shower standing up, have they considered a bath seat?

Action Items:
    a.   Place a special bathing chair in the tub. Your best choice for a bathing chair is one that will also fit in the shower.

    b.   Install a hand-held, easily reachable showerhead. These can be easier to use, especially when cleaning hard-to-reach places.

Notes:_____
_____
_____
_____
_____
_____

Safety Assessment Question: Does the elder fear getting in and/or out of the bathtub?

Action Items:
    a.   Encourage the elder to bathe only when help is available.

    b.   A family member the elder is comfortable with should be designated to be available to assist the elder with bathing.

    c.   It can be helpful to set up a schedule for bath days.

    d.   If you are assisting an elder to bathe or supervising their bathing, this can be a good time to observe their physical condition for signs of bruising, malnutrition, dehydration etc.

Notes:_____
_____
_____
_____
_____
_____

Safety Assessment Question: Are cold and hot faucets clearly marked?

    Action Item: Ensure cold and hot faucets are clearly marked.

Notes:_____
_____
_____
_____
_____
_____

Safety Assessment Question: Is the hot water temperature set to the recommended 49°C (120°F) to prevent scalding?

    Safety Assessment Question: Is a water temperature regulator present?

    Rationale: As we age, our skin becomes more sensitive to temperature changes and we can burn easier.

    Action Item: Set the hot water heater to Medium to prevent scalding.

Notes:_____
_____
_____
_____
_____
_____

Safety Assessment Question: Does the elder test the water temperature before they get into the bathtub or shower?

    Rationale: Many elders prefer warmer water than what we may prefer, so you would need to know their preferences.

Action Item: The elder should be encouraged to test the water temperature before entering.

Notes:_____
_____
_____
_____
_____
_____

Safety Assessment Question: Is the elder able to use the toilet independently and safely?

Considerations: If the elder has difficulty getting on and off the toilet, a raised toilet seat and a well-anchored grab bar can help.

Toilets should be between 17 and 19 inches in height. Seniors will find it easier to sit and stand.

Action Item: Replace the original toilet seat with a raised toilet seat with handlebars.

Notes:_____
_____
_____
_____
_____
_____

Safety Assessment Question: Are cold and hot faucets clearly marked?

Safety Assessment Question: Is there a night light in the bathroom?

Action Item: Ensure there is a night light available in the bathroom that automatically turns on in the dark.

Notes:_____
_____
_____
_____
_____
_____

Safety Assessment Question: If medication is stored in the bathroom, is it safe & secure?

Action Item: Put medicines in a lockbox and block access to cleaning supplies and razors.

Consideration: You may want to switch to a cordless electric shaver for elderly men.

Notes:_____
_____
_____
_____
_____
_____

Safety Assessment Question: Do bathroom cleaning products in use create slipperiness?

Rationale: Some tile and bath cleaning products actually increase slipperiness when applied to flooring. Be careful when using such products.

Action Item: Assess cleaning products used in the bathroom. They should not create a hazard when being used to solve a different problem.

Notes:_____
_____
_____
_____
_____
_____

Safety Assessment Question: Are bathroom cleaning products harsh or caustic?

Rationale: Harsh smelling cleaning products can create or add to existing respiratory conditions. They may trigger a breathing crisis. As bathrooms tend to be smaller rooms, especially in older homes, they don't usually provide adequate ventilation for harsh cleaning products.

Action Item: Purchase cleaning products that are safe to use, i.e. nontoxic.

Provide additional ventilation such as opening a window if it is necessary to use a harsh smelling product.

Notes:_____
_____
_____
_____
_____
_____

Safety Assessment Question: Is mildew present in the bathroom?

Rationale: We discussed mold related to food products in the chapter on kitchen safety. (See the chapter in the main book on mold.)

Action Items:

a. If the bathroom does not have an exhaust fan, it may be advisable to install one. This may require the services of a qualified electrician.

b. Wiping down a vinyl shower curtain or shower door with a dry towel after a shower can help reduce excess moisture.

Notes:_____
_____
_____
_____
_____
_____

Safety Assessment Question: Is the elder able to use the telephone? Is telephone accessible in an emergency?

Action Item: The elder should be encouraged to take a portable cordless phone into the bathroom with them in case of an emergency.

Notes:_____
_____
_____
_____
_____
_____

Safety Measures for the Bathroom:

Action Item: If the elder is showing early signs of dementia, there may be value in removing the bathroom mirror. Seeing an unfamiliar face looking back at them may be startling.

Action Items:
    a.   Install grab bars as needed. Towel racks, soap dishes or toilet paper holders should not be used for support.

    b.   Ensure there is additional lighting.

    c.   Install a nightlight in the bathroom. This will help elders who may make repeated trips to the bathroom overnight.

    d.   Install a nightlight or two on the route to the bathroom as well so elders can find their way.

    e.   Install a handheld shower head. Lever handles on faucets are recommended.

Notes:_____
_____
_____
_____

Daily activities of the elder that may increase risk:

The elder should be encouraged to wear anti-slip slippers or socks when walking around the home, especially on slippery surfaces such as polished hardwood floors or tile.

In the next chapter we assess hazards in the elder's bedroom.

Chapter Seven: Home Safety – Bedrooms

You may not think danger can lurk in an elder's bedroom, but think again! Elders can encounter several potential risks here.

Action: Do a walk about assessment

Take the **Home Safety Assessment Form** with you and do a walk about inspection of the elder's bedroom.

Safety Assessment Question: Is there a clear path from the elder's bed to the bathroom?

Considerations: If there isn't a clear path from the elder's bed to the bathroom, is it possible to rearrange the bedroom furniture to improve the route?

Action Item: If necessary, make changes to the elder's route to the bathroom from their bed.

Notes:_____
_____
_____
_____
_____
_____

Safety Assessment Question: Is there a phone and a list of emergency phone numbers near the elder's bed?

Action Items:
    a.   Create a list of emergency & frequently used numbers and place near a phone in the elder's bedroom.

    b.   Have a portable phone available which would allow the elder to carry it around the home as needed.

Notes:_____
_____
_____
_____

Safety Assessment Question: Are there night lights or other sources of light on in case the elder gets up in the middle of the night?

Rationale: Nightlights are inexpensive to purchase. A nightlight should be installed in an area that would illuminate the path to the bathroom should the elder need to visit it during the night.

Nightlights should have automatic on/off sensors.

Action Item: If an electrical outlet is not available along the path, consider purchasing a battery operated one.

Notes:_____
_____
_____
_____
_____
_____

Safety Assessment Question: Is there a lamp or a light switch near the elder's bed?

Rationale: Bedroom lamps for the elderly should have a 'touch' on/off feature rather than a push or rotating switch which can be difficult for the elderly to use.

Action Items:
    a.   Replace bedroom lamps with 'touch' on/off features.

    b.   Demonstrate to the elder how the new lamps work.

Notes:_____
_____
_____
_____
_____
_____

Safety Assessment Question: Is there a light switch near the entrance to the elder's bedroom?

Notes:_____
_____
_____
_____
_____
_____

Safety Measures:

Safety Assessment Question: Is the bed height easy for the elder to get in and out of bed?

    Make it Safe TIP: Make sure the elder's bed is not too high or low, so it is easy to get in and out of. You can purchase short bed rails to help the elder steady themselves when getting out of bed.

    Action Item: Replace a sagging, softer mattress with a firmer one. This will be far more comfortable, provide more support, and not trap a resting elder.

Notes:_____
_____
_____
_____
_____
_____

Safety Assessment Question: Assess whether door locks are required on bedroom doors to keep the elder out of other rooms or to prevent them from being locked in theirs.

    Action Item: Replace a round bedroom doorknob with a single-lever instead. An elder can easily push this lever down to open the door.

    Consideration: Consider taking the lock off the elder's door to be certain that no one is locked in or out.

    Consideration: You may want to put a lock on your own bedroom door and keep your personal and potentially dangerous items out of the elder's reach.

Notes:_____
_____
_____
_____
_____
_____

Safety Devices:

Audio monitor: An audio monitor between the two rooms will let you hear if the elder is out of bed or calling for help.

Action Item: If the elder has mobility challenges, getting in and out of bed can be a problem for them. Fit the bedroom with a telescoping grab bar that extends between the floor and ceiling. This can assist the elder with mobility problems in getting in or out of bed independently.

Notes:_____
_____
_____
_____
_____
_____

∼

In the next chapter we assess hazards located in the outdoors surrounding an elder's home.

Chapter Eight: Home Safety - The Great Outdoors

The outdoors isn't necessarily great if it presents a risk for your elder to enjoy. If you live in an area that has four distinct seasons, each season can bring its own risk.

Action Item: Take the **Home Safety Assessment Form** with you and do a walk about inspection of the outside of the elder's home.

Safety Assessment Question: Do all entrances have an outdoor light?

Action Item: Ensure pathways and steps have adequate lighting.

Notes:_____
_____
_____
_____
_____
_____

Safety Assessment Question: Do the doorways to your balcony or deck have a low sill or threshold?

Action Item: If possible, add a wedge or a new threshold to prevent tripping.

Consideration: Consider painting the repair so the elder can see it better.

Notes:_____
_____
_____
_____
_____
_____

Safety Assessment Question: Are there solid handrails on both sides of an outdoor stairway?

As we discussed earlier in our chapter on Home Safety - Hallways & Stairwells...

Action Item: If stair railings <u>are</u> present, test them for stability.

Rationale: You don't have to be a home handyman to do this. Grab the railing and try to shake it back and forth. If the railing wiggles (even somewhat), it's time to fix it. Tighten all nuts and bolts or replace the railing.

Action Item: If solid handrails <u>are not</u> present on outdoor stairways, install them on both sides of the stairs. This may require a skilled tradesperson to install the handrails.

Notes:_____
_____
_____
_____
_____
_____
_____

Safety Assessment Question: Do outdoor steps and thresholds cause a hazard for elderly residents?

Action Item: Assess outdoor steps for safety.

Notes:_____
_____
_____
_____
_____
_____
_____

Safety Assessment Question: Are there stairs outside of the home the elder must navigate to enter/exit the home?

Considerations: If the elder has mobility problems, explore the possibility of installing a mechanical stair lift which can smoothly carry your loved one up or down a flight of stairs.

Alternatively, consider if a wheelchair ramp can be placed at the front side or rear of the home. If land space is limited know that a wheelchair ramp does not have to extend straight out it can be built to a double back on itself or even curled around. Ensure the incline is not too steep and the ramp features secure handrails your parents can pull himself up if need be.

Action Items:
   a. Determine if a mechanical stair lift or wheelchair ramp is feasible.

b. Research the costs involved with either initiative.

c. Create a budget if viable.

d. Research to see if any funding is available to offset costs of the renovation.

Notes:_____
_____
_____
_____
_____
_____
_____

Safety Assessment Question: Look at access to decks and porch areas. Is there a step to the patio? Is there a sliding door threshold to step over?

Action Item: See previous Assessment question above re steps and thresholds.

Notes:_____
_____
_____
_____
_____
_____
_____

Safety Assessment Question: Can the elder reach their mailbox safely and easily?

Action Item: Assess the mailbox for height. If the elder is unable to retrieve their mail due to an inappropriate height for them, adjust as needed.

Notes:_____
_____
_____
_____
_____
_____
_____

Safety Assessment Question: Is the number of the house clearly visible from the street and well-lit at night?

Action Item: Ensure the home address is visible during the day or night.

Make it Safe TIP: If you live in a rural area and don't have a visible house number, make sure your name is on your mailbox and keep a clear description of directions to your home (main roads, landmarks, etc.) by each phone in your house.

Make it Safe TIP: Some fire departments provide highly reflective address numbers at low to no cost or they can be purchased on-line.

Notes:_____
_____
_____
_____
_____
_____

Neighborhood Risks:

Safety Assessment Question: Are there any risks inherent to the neighborhood of the elder's home?

Action Item: Create a list of possible hazards in the neighborhood that could cause problems for an elder. Example: heavy traffic, busy intersections, schools, shops, etc.

Notes:_____
_____
_____
_____
_____
_____

Remain safe in the home:

Action Item: Review common sense safety measures with your elder.

Rationale: It can be tempting to open the door to someone who "looks nice" but beware.

Here are some other **action items** for you to do and to remind them about:

    a.   Install a peephole in your senior's front door.

b. Do not open the door to strangers when home alone.

c. Place a reminder note on the wall beside the front door saying, "Do you know this person? If not, do not open the door."

d. Always keep windows and doors locked.

e. Install a mail slot in the front door to prevent mail theft.

Notes:_____
_____
_____
_____
_____
_____
_____

Safety Assessment Question: Is the home safe for a professional caregiver to visit the home?

Rationale: Professional caregivers are trained to consider their own health and safety first. If the home presents a potential hazard to their personal safety, they may deny service until the hazard has been rectified.

Action Item: Correct or remove any hazards that would prevent a professional care giver from visiting the elder's home.

Notes:_____
_____
_____
_____
_____
_____
_____

Safety Assessment Question: Is there patio furniture that would cause problems for an elder to get in and out of?

Considerations: Be cautious of patio furniture as it can be low and difficult for seniors to transfer into or out of.

Action Items:

      a.   Remove and replace patio furniture that is too low for elders to easily get in and out of.

      b.   Discard patio furniture that is broken or in need of repair.

Notes:_____
_____
_____
_____
_____
_____

Safety Assessment Question: Are there any damaged steps or cracks in outdoor sidewalks?

Considerations: Walking on grass can be difficult for older adults with mobility issues.

Action Items:
      a.   Check to see if there are paved paths to access gardens or backyards.

      b.   Secure and repair uneven walkways or patio stones.

      c.   Repair damaged steps or cracks in outdoor sidewalks.

Notes:_____
_____
_____
_____
_____
_____

Safety Assessment Question: Are there any hazards such as leaves and ice on outside pathways?

Action Items:
      a.   Keep walkways and patios clear of fallen leaves and branches, ice and snow.

      b.   Corral any toys.

      c.   Remove hazards such as leaves and ice from outside pathways.

Notes:_____
_____
_____
_____
_____
_____

Safety Assessment Question: Does the elder use a motorized scooter?

> **Considerations:** If so, do they use it safely?
> Have they been trained in its safe use?
> Who maintains it?

Notes:_____
_____
_____
_____
_____
_____

Safety Assessment Question: Are emergency plans in place such as leaving a key with a neighbor in the case of the elder being locked out?

> **Action Items:**
> a. Leave a key with a neighbor you trust, in case the elder is locked out.
> b. Remind the elder who has a spare key in case they are locked out.

Notes:_____
_____
_____
_____
_____
_____

Safety Assessment Question: Are BBQ grills locked & covered when not in use?

> **Action Item:** Keep the grill locked and covered when not in use.

Notes:_____
_____
_____
_____
_____
_____

Safety Assessment Question: If you live in an area that has seasonal snow falls, are there plans in place for timely snow removal?

Rationale: Studies have shown those aged above 55 should not shovel snow. A research team discovered that even with healthy young men, shoveling snow showed a great impact on their physical state – their heart rate and blood pressure increased more than when they exercised on a treadmill.

Combine this with cold air, which causes arteries to constrict and decrease blood supply, and you have a perfect storm for a heart attack.

Source: Country Living
https://www.countryliving.com/uk/wellbeing/news/a3030/shovelling-snow-heart-attack-risk/

Action Item: Assuming you are well under 55 years old, capable and available to shovel the elder's driveway and sidewalk, do so.
If not, hire someone to shovel the snow when required.

Notes:_____
_____
_____
_____
_____
_____

Miscellaneous Outdoor Safety Devices:

Outdoor motion lights:

Action Item: Install outdoor motion sensor lights and path lights to help the elder see after dark.

Notes:_____
_____
_____
_____
_____
_____

Fenced-in yard:

Action Item: A fenced-in yard will allow the elder to go outside. Make sure gates lock.

Notes:_____
_____
_____
_____
_____
_____

Pool Safety:

Automatic pool cover:

Action Item: Consider installing an automatic rolling pool cover that is made to withstand the weight of people and lock in place. Use the cover whenever the pool is not monitored by someone capable of rescuing a non-swimmer-- even if you'll just be gone a few minutes.

Notes:_____
_____
_____
_____
_____
_____

Pool alarm:

Action Item: Use a pool alarm with an electric sensor that will trip a loud, pulsating alarm -- outside and in the house -- when anyone enters the water. The alarm uses an on-off key.

Notes:_____
_____
_____
_____
_____
_____

Pull-up pool ladder:

Action Item: If you have an above-ground pool, a pull-up and locking ladder is a must. Make sure it is properly installed.

Notes:_____
_____
_____
_____
_____
_____

Daily activities of the elder that may increase risk:

Safety Assessment Question: Does the elder smoke outside?

Action Items:
    a.   If so, provide a designated safe and protected from the elements area for the elder to smoke.

    b.   Fire and wind proof ashtrays should be supplied for outside smoking.

    c.   Ashtrays should be cleaned and emptied on a regular basis.

Notes:_____
_____
_____
_____

∼

In the next chapter we look at safety hazards related to home use medical devices.

Home Use Medical Devices

As a homecare medical device user, you should know how your device works.
Action Items:

    a.   Read your patient education information.

    b.   Ask your doctor or supplier questions about your device, and take notes.

    c.   Ask what you need to operate your device.

    d.   Do you need electricity, running water, telephone, or computer connections to operate your device?

    e.   Check to see that your home is suited for your device.

    f.   Do the stairs, doorways, bathrooms, house wiring present any problems?

    g.   Keep <u>Instructions for Use</u> close to your device.

    h.   Pay attention to alarms and error messages.

    i.   Be familiar with what the alarms and error messages mean.

    j.   Follow Instructions as given.

    k.   Call supplier for help if you don't understand how your device works.

    l.   Report to your doctor or device supplier any new problems you have with the device.

Take care of your device and operate it according to the manufacturer's directions.
Action Items:

a. Read your instructions for taking care of your device and follow them for:

- Cleaning
- replacing batteries, filters
- protecting your device (e.g. keep food and drinks away from your device).

b. Can you safely take your device from home to school, work, church, and vacation spots?

c. Check ahead to see if these other places are suited for your device.

d. Dispose of your medical device according to the manufacturer's instructions.

e. Always have a back-up plan and supplies.

f. Make sure you know what to do if your device fails.

g. Have emergency phone numbers for suppliers, homecare agency, doctor, and manufacturer.

h. Be sure that you have the after-hour phone numbers.

i. If appropriate, keep extra batteries for your device.

j. Know how to replace them.

k. Educate your family and caregivers about your devices:
- Include them in hospital planning meetings or any device demonstrations.
- Ask them to do a hands-on demonstration to show they can effectively use the device.
- Keep children and pets away from your medical device.
- Don't let children play with dials, Settings, on/off switches, tubings, machine vents, or electrical cords.

l. Don't allow pets to chew or play with electrical cords.
m. Check with your supplier to see if you can turn off your device when not using it.

Contact your doctor and home healthcare team often to review your health condition.
a. Check to see if there are new conditions that may change the way you or your caregiver use the device.
b. Are there changes in vision, hearing, ability to move?
c. Have you had an illness, new medicines, loss of feeling?

Notes:_____
_____
_____
_____

In the next chapter we look at electrical safety hazards and how to avoid them.

Chapter Nine: Electrical Safety

In this chapter we feature questions, tips and action items related to electrical safety, gathered from the previous chapters for an easy, quick reference and expand upon them where necessary.

If you or your elder live in an older home, it would be wise to have a qualified electrician inspect the house's wiring, fuse box, electrical cords and appliances for safety.

The money you spend on an electrical safety inspection could provide you with some much-needed peace of mind.

Let's start off with assessing the home's lighting.

Rationale: Aging eyes don't always work as they once did. Elders may misjudge or completely avoid darkened areas in their home.

Action Items:

a. Locate and replace any burnt-out light bulbs. Consider substituting the newer lower power consuming and brighter LED bulbs.

b. Test all lighting for effectiveness by standing in one corner of a room and looking across the room. Can you see a clear path? If not, brighten things up with more lights.

c. Install new light fixtures where needed.

d. Install motion detection lighting inside and outside the home.

Rationale: Motion activated indoor lighting is available in hard-wired and battery-operated versions. The battery-operated versions can be an ideal solution in areas where installing an electrical fixture isn't practical or is cost prohibitive.

Notes:_____
_____
_____
_____
_____

Safety Assessment Question: Is there good lighting in stairways & hallways?

    Action Item: Provide effective lighting where required.
Make home lighting brighter but prevent glare.

Notes:_____
_____
_____
_____
_____
_____
_____

Safety Assessment Question: Does every room have proper lighting, including walk-in closets?

    Action Item: Ensure every room has proper lighting, including walk-in closets. Use a nightlight to make it easy to see at night. Battery operated nightlights are available for areas without electrical access.

Notes:_____
_____
_____
_____
_____
_____
_____

Safety Assessment Question: Is there a lamp or a light switch near the elder's bed?

    Action Item: Place a light (such as a lamp) close to the bed and make sure the elder can reach it easily.

    Bedroom lamps for the elderly should have a 'touch' on/off feature rather than a push or rotating switch which can be difficult for the elderly to use.

    Extra lamps-- consider models that turn on and off with a touch of the hand.

Notes:_____
_____
_____
_____
_____
_____

Safety Assessment Question: Are there light switches at the top and bottom of your staircases and/or hallways?

Action Item: Install light switches at the top and bottom of your staircases. This installation would require the services of a qualified electrician.

Notes:_____
_____
_____
_____
_____
_____

Safety Assessment Question: Is there adequate lighting for safely moving in the hallway or stairwell?

Rationale: The existing light fixtures may be adequate if a suitable light bulb is installed. There are a variety of lightbulbs e.g. halogen and LED that provide more light, last longer, shed less heat and are more economical to operate.

If good lighting is not present e.g. inappropriately placed, it may be necessary to contact a qualified electrician to install additional light fixture(s).

Action Item: Ensure there is good lighting in stairways and hallways.

Notes:_____
_____
_____
_____
_____
_____

Safety Assessment Question: Are there night lights or other sources of light in case the elder gets up in the middle of the night?

Rationale: Night-lights are inexpensive to purchase. A nightlight should be installed in an area that would illuminate the path to the bathroom should the elder need to visit it during the night.

If an electrical outlet is not available along the path, consider purchasing a battery operated one.

Night-lights should have automatic on/off sensors.

Action Item: If lighting is not adequate, install new light fixtures along the path between the bathroom and the elder's bedroom.

Notes:_____
_____
_____
_____
_____
_____

Safety Assessment Questions: Is there a light switch near the entrance to the elder's bedroom? & Is there a night light in the bathroom?

Action Items:
a. Ensure there is a night light available in the bathroom that automatically comes on in the dark. This will help elders who may make repeated trips to the bathroom overnight.

b. Ensure that there is additional lighting. Install a nightlight or two on the route to the bathroom as well so that elders can find their way.

Notes:_____
_____
_____
_____
_____
_____

Safety Assessment Question: Are controls & switches reachable from a wheelchair or bed?

If possible, are you able to relocate controls and switches so they are reachable from a wheelchair or bed?

Notes:_____
_____

Electrical Outlets, Power Bars & Extension Cords

Safety Assessment Question: Are electrical outlets or power bars overloaded or used unsafely e.g. daisy-chained?

Rationale: Daisy chaining is where one power bar or extension cord is plugged into another one and possibly even another.

Do not overload power sockets or extension cords.

Action Item: If any of the appliance power cords or wires are torn or frayed, replace them immediately to decrease the risk of fire.

If power cords or extension cords are necessary, purchase ones rated for the energy they are expected to carry and for the correct length.

Notes:_____
_____
_____
_____
_____
_____

Safety Assessment Question: Are electrical cords or cables exposed in a way that could be a trip hazard?

Action Item: Avoid stretching extension cords across the floor.

Notes:_____
_____
_____
_____
_____
_____

Appliance Safety-- Large and Small Appliances

Action Item: Have a professional or plumber clean the vents of your dryer once every three months. Dryer vents cause 2,900 fires every year (USA), and the leading cause of these fires is failure to clean them.

Don't leave your dryer running when you are sleeping, or not at home.

Notes:_____
_____
_____
_____
_____
_____

Safety Assessment Question: Are appliance cords in good condition?

Action Items: Service your appliances every 3-6 months.

Rationale: Many seniors keep important medication in their refrigerators, so it's important to make sure they are in good working condition. If you have a clothes dryer, make sure the vents are cleaned by a professional, to prevent risk of fire.

If any appliance power cords or wires are torn or frayed, replace them immediately to decrease the risk of fire.

Notes:_____
_____
_____
_____
_____
_____

Electrical Safety Devices for the kitchen:

Safety Assessment Question: Is an automatic stove shut off device in place?

Considerations: Consider using automatic devices to turn off the stove and oven or installing an induction cooktop -- which turns off when a pot is removed from the burner.

Automatic shutoffs on small appliances are recommended.

Action Item: Install an automatic device to turn off the stove after a set period if no movement is detected.

Notes:_____
_____
_____
_____
_____
_____

Electrical Safety Devices for the Bathroom:

Safety Assessment Questions: Are all electrical outlets in the bathroom GFCIs and are they tested regularly?

Action Item: Ensure outlets in the bathroom have a ground fault circuit interrupter (GFCI) or are protected by a GFCI circuit so it will close the circuit should a person with wet hands come in contact with the receptacle.

Notes:_____
_____
_____
_____
_____
_____

Home Heating:

Safety Assessment Question: Does the home have an adequate heating system or does the elder use the stove or oven to provide heat?

Action Items:

    a.   Heat the home safely – do not use an oven as a heating source, under any circumstance.

    b.   Turn off all portable heaters when you leave your home.

Notes:_____
_____
_____
_____
_____
_____

Safety Assessment Question: If the elder uses a space heater, is it placed well away from flammable substances and materials?

Action Item: Ensure all electrical equipment around the house works properly. This includes air conditioning units – seniors are at higher risk of adverse effects due to high temperatures.

Notes:_____
_____
_____
_____
_____
_____

We look at fire safety in greater depth in the next chapter.

Chapter Ten: Fire Safety & Prevention

We've mentioned fire prevention and safety measures in other chapters as we've moved around the house.

This chapter summarizes and expands upon those preventative actions.

Safety Assessment Question: Have you developed an escape route in case of fire and a fire safety plan?

Rationale: Decreased mobility, sight, hearing or cognitive capabilities may limit a person's ability to take the quick action necessary to escape during a fire emergency. People over the age of 65 are twice as likely to suffer injuries or lose their lives in fires compared to the population-at-large, according to the U.S. Fire Administration, part of the Federal Emergency Management Agency (FEMA).

If you are caring for someone with Alzheimer's or dementia, problems with mobility, or if vision or hearing impaired, there are certain precautions that need to be taken in the event of a house fire. These precautions go above and beyond the traditional fire safety guidelines for all families.

Action Items:

a. Check all exits to make sure wheelchairs or walkers can get through the doorways. Make any necessary accommodations (such as installation of exit ramps) to facilitate an emergency escape.

b. Install flooring material that accommodates artificial limbs or canes.

c. Keep a phone by the bed for emergency calls in case the person becomes trapped and is unable to escape. Put emergency numbers in the speed dial directory of the phone.

d. People confined to a wheelchair may want to have a small 'personal use' fire extinguisher mounted in an accessible place on the wheelchair and become familiar with its use.

e. When escape is not an option due to impaired mobility, fire protection devices such as sprinkler systems, fire-safe compartment walls, and flame-resistant blankets can be used. The key is to have the room fireproofed before an emergency happens.

f. Remain calm during an emergency. Explain what is happening clearly and simply, but don't expect them to remember specific details. Validate their concerns, but provide clear direction without condescending or losing patience.

g. Provide a picture book of emergency procedures. A cognitively impaired person may be able to follow visual instructions more easily. Contact your local fire department or the National Fire Protection agency.

h. Practice escape routes. Cognition tends to improve and worsen at various times for people with Alzheimer's or dementia. If escape is practiced continually, instinct may take over and guide the elder to safety.

i. The person should sleep in a room that has easy access to the outdoors in case the home needs to be evacuated. A ground floor bedroom is best.

Action Items:
a. Give due consideration to the advice offered above and apply it to your situation.

b. Work with your elder to develop an emergency escape plan that works for them. If the elder lives in your home with you or your family, don't forget to develop an escape route for yourselves.

c. If the elder's home is in an apartment building, are they registered on the apartment building's fire safety plan?

Notes:_____
_____
_____
_____
_____
_____

Safety Assessment Question: If the elder uses a portable space heater, is it placed well away from flammable substances and materials?

Safety Assessment Question: If the elder uses a portable space heater, is it plugged into the wall or to an extension cord/power bar?

Rationale: According to Mr. Google... space heaters are behind 79 percent of deadly home heating fires, according to the National Fire Protection Association. Half of those fires start because an object sitting within three feet of the heater got too hot and caught fire, but even plugging the equipment into the wrong outlet could put you in danger.

Cheap power strips shouldn't be used for anything that needs to stay plugged in for long periods of time because they don't have surge protectors. Because they have so much start up energy and because they heat up so quickly and for such a prolonged time, the heat transference goes back down to the power strip and causes it to overheat.

Action Item: Assess whether a portable space heater, if used, is being used safely.

Rationale: Again... from Mr. Google... do not plug any other electrical devices into the same outlet as the heater. Place space heaters on level, flat surfaces. Never place heaters on cabinets, tables, furniture, or carpet, which can overheat and start a fire. Always unplug and safely store the heater when it is not in use.

Considerations: Why is the portable space heater even being used?
- Is the home's heating system providing sufficient heat?
- Are there cold zones in the house where the elder feels the need to provide additional heat?
- If a portable space heater is being used, is it safe?
- Is the electrical cord frayed or in good condition?
- If a portable space heater is deemed necessary, is this the most appropriate one available?
- Does the portable space heater have safety features to prevent fire?

Examples:

Overheat Protection: Room heaters with overheat protection detect when internal components become too hot. When an unsafe temperature is detected, the switch automatically shuts off the unit to prevent overheating.

Tip-Over Protection: A heater equipped with a tip-over protection switch will automatically shut off if it's tipped over for any reason.

Cool-Touch Housing: Cool-touch housing prevents accidental burns by touching the exterior of a heater. This is particularly useful safety feature, particularly in areas with active children or pets.

Action Item: If a portable space heater is in use, provide regular inspection and maintenance.

Occasionally inspect your portable space heater, particularly when you first purchase it. Frequently clean and maintain it to ensure it's working safely.

Wiping yours down will also help reduce the amount of dust and allergens that may be dispersed around your space.

Encourage the elder to unplug the portable space heater when it's not in use.

More Considerations: Keep portable heaters away from water.

Unless it is specifically designed for use in damp spaces, refrain from running a heater in a bathroom or a humid basement. Don't touch the heater if you are wet or have wet hands, as this increases the risk of electrical shock.

Notes:_____
_____
_____
_____
_____
_____

Prevent Poisoning: Carbon Monoxide

Make it Safe TIP:
- Never try to heat your home with your stove, oven, or grill since these can give off carbon monoxide-- a deadly gas that you cannot see or smell.
- Make sure there is a carbon monoxide detector near all bedrooms and be sure to test and replace the battery two times a year.

Safety Assessment Question: If the home is older, have you or an electrician inspected the house wiring, fuse box, electrical cords and appliances for safety?

Action Item: Have a professional or plumber clean the vents of your dryer once every three months. Dryer vents cause 2,900 fires every year (USA), and the leading cause of these fires is failure to clean them.

Notes:_____
_____
_____
_____
_____
_____

Safety Assessment Question: If the elder cooks, do they practice safe cooking techniques?

Hazard: Leaving the stove unattended or cooking at too high heat.

Rationale: One in five Americans admits to leaving food cooking unattended on the stove, found an American Red Cross survey. Walking away from food cooking in the kitchen is a serious fire risk. "The leading cause of home fires is cooking, and the leading cause of those fires is unattended cooking."

Notes:_____
_____
_____
_____
_____
_____

Safety Assessment Question: Does your elder smoke?

Hazard: Not fully extinguishing cigarettes.

While cooking is the leading cause of home fires, smoking is actually the leading cause of home fire deaths. If you have people in your home who smoke, make sure they smoke outside and extinguish all their cigarettes completely in sand or water.

Source: Readers Digest https://www.rd.com/home/improvement/fire-hazards-in-home/

Considerations: If the elder lives with you in your own home, you can set restrictions where the elder can and cannot smoke.

If the elder lives in their own home, you may not be successful in setting smoking restrictions. Long-time smokers can be very set in their ways and can become defensive when limitations are set upon them. Smoking is an addiction and addictive habits have a way of trying to protect the individual from going through withdrawal.

Action Items:
    a.   The elder should be encouraged to quit smoking for health and safety reasons. At the very least, cutting down on the frequency of smoking can help.

    b.   The elder should be encouraged to smoke in a designated area, outside.

  c. Fire and wind proof ashtrays should be supplied for outside smoking.

  d. Ashtrays should be cleaned and emptied on a regular basis.

Notes:_____
_____
_____
_____
_____
_____

Safety Assessment Question: Does the elder drink alcohol?

Do they drink to excess and increase the potential for hazard? i.e. to themselves or the home?

Considerations: Drinking alcoholic beverages is considered by many people to be one of the perks and pleasures of being an adult. A daily alcoholic drink may be the elder's only pleasure in life. Not my words... but I've heard it many times.

On the other hand, an elder with alcoholism may increase the level of risk.

Action Items:
  a. Assess the situation for degree of risk.

  b. Develop safety measures to reduce the risk. Examples: only allowing smoking in designated areas outside, etc.

Notes:_____
_____
_____
_____
_____
_____

Safety Assessment Question: Are flammable and hazardous materials clearly labeled and properly stored? Is there a designated danger zone in the home to store hazardous chemicals or products?

Rationale: We discussed creating a designated area or danger zone in our previous chapter on Home Safety - Indoors General. The same principles apply to flammable and hazardous materials.

Action Item: Designate a danger zone or remove a hazardous product from the household.

Examples of hazardous products: lighter fluid, barbecue starter fluid, gasoline, portable appliance fuel e.g. butane or propane for hair dryers, kerosene, etc.

Notes:_____
_____
_____
_____
_____
_____

General Fire Prevention Safety Measures

Change the batteries in smoke and carbon monoxide detectors regularly (after seasonal time changes).

Check the electric cords of all appliances and lamps in your loved one's home. Replace any frayed or damaged cords and limit the number of cords plugged into power strips.

Remove candles from the home. If left burning and unattended, candles can start a fire.

Remind seniors to stay low when exiting the home in a fire. This reduces the chance of smoke inhalation. Coach seniors on how to "stop, drop, and roll" if their clothes ignite.

Discourage the use of portable space heaters. If your loved one insists on using one, place it at least three feet away from curtains, bedding, or furniture. Remind your loved one to turn off the portable space heater before going to bed or leaving the house.

In our next chapter we look at what you need to do after you've completed your home safety assessment and what you should be looking for on subsequent visits to the elder's home.

This page has been intentionally left blank.

Chapter Eleven: Ongoing Follow-up

Home safety for elders means checking in with them regularly.

Do you live in the same town or city as the elder you are supporting? Drop in unannounced to get a better idea of how they are truthfully doing. If you don't live close to the elder, arrange with someone else to take on the responsibility of ongoing follow-up.

Considerations: By now you have probably realized how much time and effort is involved in supporting an elder living semi-independently in the community. It can be a little easier, in some ways, when the elder is living in your home with you.

For those elders living semi-independent there may be value in arranging for a maid/cleaning service to visit the elder's home once a week for light housekeeping duties. This would include dusting, vacuuming and cleaning untidy areas of the home. Kitchens and bathrooms often require extra attention.

Several times a year, perhaps quarterly, a deeper cleaning could be organized to include cleaning the windows, vacuuming areas that wouldn't have been done in the regular cleaning e.g. Overhead ceiling fan's blades, behind furniture, walls and ceilings, etc.

This, in turn, can take a lot of pressure off you.

Action Items:

    a.   Be on the lookout for anything that has changed or needs repaired since your last visit.

    b.   Ask the elder if there is anything broken or needing fixing.

    c.   Check the kitchen stove/cooktop grease filters to see if they need cleaning.

    d.   Check on the home's indoor temperature. Is it appropriate compared to the outdoor temperature?. Examples: warm in the winter and cooler in the summer if hot outdoors.

    e.   Is the elder wearing clothing appropriate for the weather conditions?

    f.   Monitor an elder in extreme hot or cold weather (when the risk of heat stroke or frostbite is higher).

    g.   Advise the elder to call you for help before trying to tackle a cleaning or repair job independently.

h. While visiting make a list of areas that need tidying and create a list of cleaning supplies that may need to be purchased. If you have the time, clean the area. If not, schedule a time to return and complete the cleaning.

i. Check portable phones for its charge. Replace a low charge phone with a fully charged one from the phone charger.

j. Remind an elder to move more slowly from one room to the next – there is often no reason to rush.

k. Keep a close eye on permanent fixtures that can become hazards -- including garbage disposals, ovens, stove tops and gas fireplaces.

l. Ensure emergency contact phone numbers remain posted in a central location such as the elder's refrigerator.

m. Check the refrigerator for signs of food spoilage and expiry dates on food containers.

n. If the elder is a smoker, look for signs of burns on furniture and clothing from cigarettes.

o. Observe the elder for any visible signs of cuts or bruising, which could be indicative of the elder tripping or falling.

p. Observe the elder's home for signs of clutter build up or new hazards that may have developed.

q. If you are supporting an elder who is living semi-independently, set up a regular shopping day with them.

r. Help them develop a shopping list in advance. [Many caregivers find this to be a frustrating task, as the elder tends to want to shop for something when they think of it, not waiting until the designated shopping day.

s. This can result in frequent requests of the caregiver to take the elder shopping which can impinge upon the caregiver's ability to manage their own time.]

t. Stock their pantry with healthy snacks (e.g. yogurt, granola bars, nuts, cheese and crackers, and fruit).

CONCLUSION

Congratulations for making it to the end of this workbook.

I would expect you have discovered many more potential hazards you hadn't considered when you started the home assessment process.

Creating this book and the original Elder Safety session in the Elder@Home Program has been an eye-opener for me as well.

While working in healthcare I found I had a different degree of control over my environment. If I noticed a hazard, I was in a position to either fix it myself or report it and have somebody else responsible for maintenance resolve the problem. Sometimes, it didn't always get fixed as fast as I would have liked.

It's not quite the same at home. It can be easy to get complacent when you're looking at something you see every day that could develop into a hazard. Procrastination can set in with the attitude of "I'll fix that someday."

At 65 years of age when writing this book, I consider myself a senior rather than an elder. The clock is ticking as it is for everyone and my elder days are approaching.

Now that I am retired, I have the time to make those household safety improvements as *"someday"* has arrived for me.

I'm hoping to live in this home for another 10 or 15 years. The safety improvements I make will go a long way in allowing that to happen.

Now the big question is, what are you going to do about it?

If you have read this book, start to finish, without completing the assessment for the elder's home, now's the time to do it.

This can be a daunting task. We covered a lot of different areas throughout the book.
I'm reminded of an old adage that goes "how do you eat an elephant?"

Answer… not that I would ever even consider eating an elephant, the answer is "one bite at a time."

Applying that principle, you may want to focus on one area of the home at a time for your assessment. This will allow you to focus on any hazards you identified and create an action plan you can realistically follow through with. As mentioned in the book, not every problem or hazard can be resolved easily or quickly.

Solving a problem may require a budget. Finding the money for the fix can be a challenge. Will you pay for it out of your pocket or can you have the elder reimburse you for your expenses? This process can take time.

Getting back to the concept of one bite at a time, once you have completed your assessment of a specific area, move on to another area of the home with your assessment.

In conclusion, I would like to thank you for your interest in your caring to support an elder. As I mentioned in the beginning of the book, it takes a family to support an elder to live as independently as they can, for as long as they can.

Rae A. Stonehouse

CONNECT WITH US

Visit us on the web at https://elderathome.ca

Follow us on Facebook (https://www.facebook.com/agingwithhelp) for a source of informational, thought-provoking articles to help you in your role as a family caregiver.

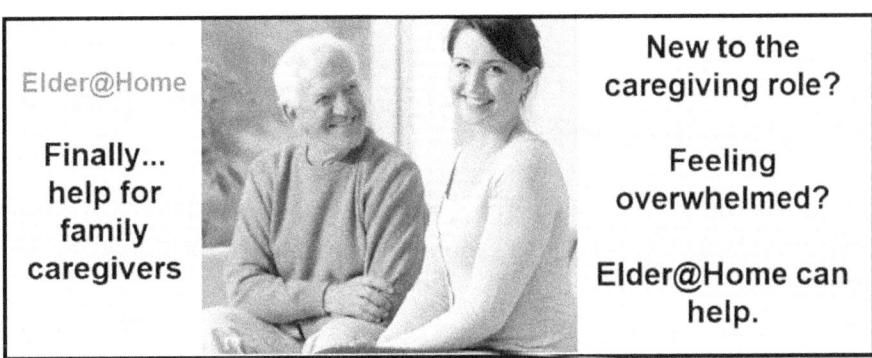

The main book Make It Safe! A Family Caregiver's Home Safety Assessment Guide is available for immediately download as an e-book at https://makeitsafe.online and in paperback at the same address.

ABOUT THE AUTHOR

Rae A. Stonehouse is a Canadian born author & speaker.

His professional career as a Registered Nurse working predominantly in psychiatry/mental health, has spanned four decades.

Rae has embraced the principal of CANI (Constant and Never-ending Improvement) as promoted by thought leaders such as Tony Robbins and brings that philosophy to each of his publications and presentations.

Rae has dedicated the latter segment of his journey through life to overcoming his personal inhibitions. As a 25+ year member of Toastmasters International he has systematically built his self-confidence and communicating ability.

He is passionate about sharing his lessons with his readers and listeners.

His publications thus far are of the self-help, self-improvement genre and systematically offer valuable sage advice on a specific topic.

His writing style can be described as being conversational. As an author Rae strives to have a one-to-one conversation with each of his readers, very much like having your own personal self-development coach.

Rae is known for having a wry sense of humour that features in his publications. To learn more about Rae A. Stonehouse, **visit The Wonderful World of Rae Stonehouse** at https://raestonehouse.com

Facebook: https://www.facebook.com/raestonehouse.aws

Twitter: https://twitter.com/raestonehouse

ALSO BY RAE A. STONEHOUSE

PROtect Yourself! Empowering Tips & Techniques for Personal Safety: A Practical Violence Prevention Manual for Healthcare Workers https://books2read.com/protectyourself

∼

Power of Promotion: On-line Marketing for Toastmasters Club Growth

https://books2read.com/powerofpromotion

∼

You're Hired! Job Search Strategies That Work (This is the complete program)

E-book & Paperback: https://yourehirednow.com

On-line E-course: (Available as a self-directed or instructor-led program) https://liveforexcellenceacademy.com/

∼

You're Hired! Resume Tactics: Job Search Strategies That Work

E-book & Paperback: https://resumetactics.online

On-line E-course: https://liveforexcellenceacademy.com/

∼

Job Interview Preparation: Job Search Strategies That Work

E-book & Paperback: https://jobinterviewpreparation.online/

On-line E-course: https://liveforexcellenceacademy.com/

∼

You're Hired! Leveraging Your Network: Job Search Strategies That Work

E-book & Paperback: https://leveragingyournetwork.online/

On-line E-course: https://liveforexcellenceacademy.com/

∽

You're Hired! Power Tactics: Job Search Strategies That Work

(This is an e-box set containing the complete content of Resume Tactics, Job Interview Preparation & Leveraging Your Network)

E-book: https://powertactics.online/

∽

Power Networking for Shy People: How to Network Like a Pro

E-book & Paperback: https://powernetworkingforshypeople.ca

∽

The Savvy Emcee: How to be a Dynamic Master of Ceremonies

E-book: https://thesavvyemcee.com

∽

Working With Words: How to Add Life to Your Oral Presentations

E-book & Paperback: https://workingwithwordsbook.com/

Also available as an on-line course at https://liveforexcellenceacademy.com

∽

Blow Your Own Horn! Personal Branding for Business Professionals

E-book & Paperback: https://blowyourownhorn.online/

～

If you have found this book and program to be helpful, please leave us a warm review wherever you purchased this book.

www.ingramcontent.com/pod-product-compliance
Lightning Source LLC
Chambersburg PA
CBHW081508080526
44589CB00017B/2688